The Social and Psychological Origins of the Climacteric Syndrome

For Elisabeth and the children

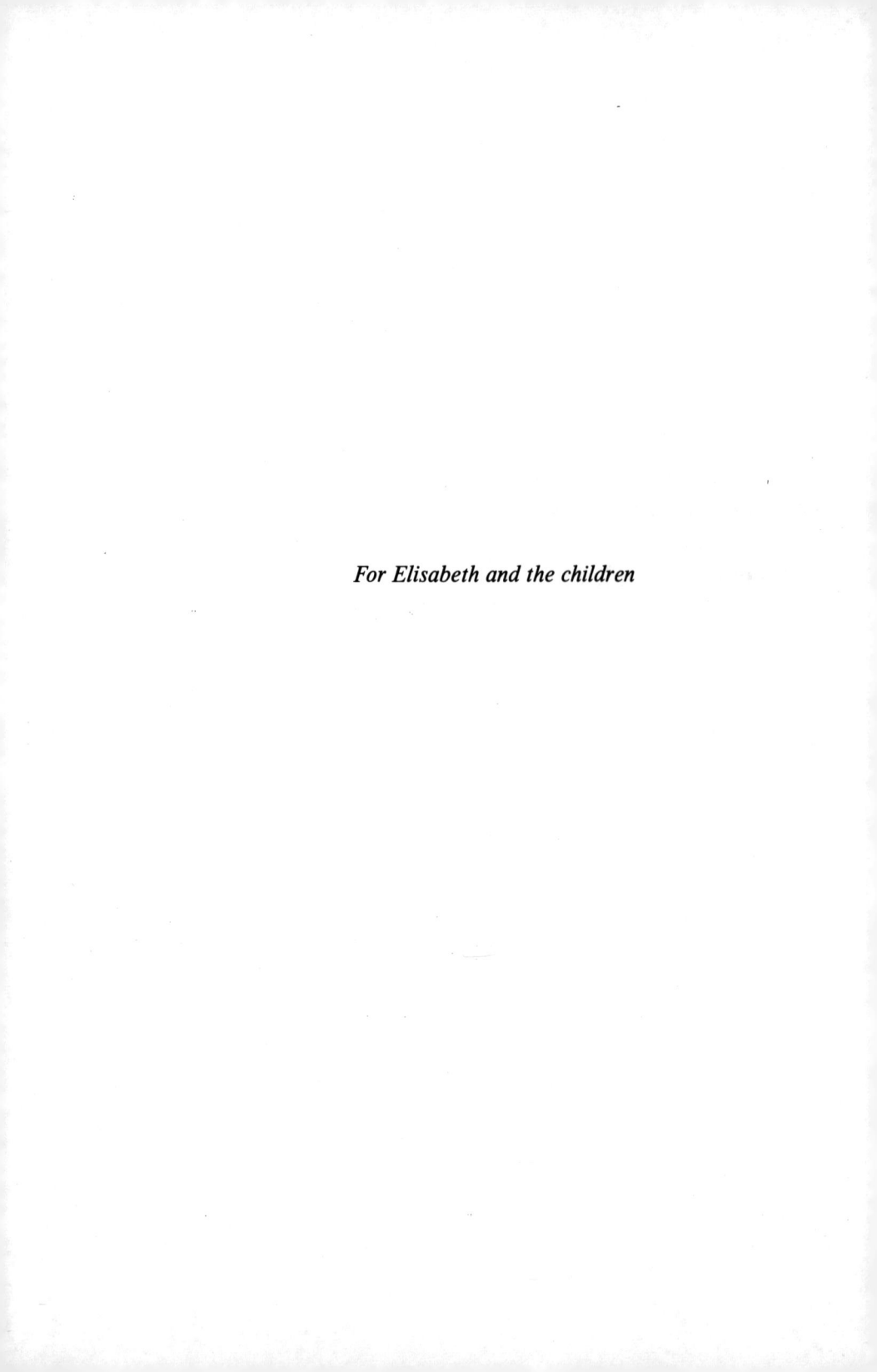

John Gerald Greene

The Social and Psychological Origins of the Climacteric Syndrome

Gower

© J.G. Greene, 1984

All rights reserved. No part of this publication may be reproduced, stored in a retrieval system, or transmitted in any form or by any means, electronic, mechanical, photocopying, recording, or otherwise without the prior permission of Gower Publishing Company Limited.

Published by
Gower Publishing Company Limited,
Gower House,
Croft Road,
Aldershot,
Hants GU11 3HR
England

and

Gower Publishing Company,
Old Post Road,
Brookfield,
Vermont 05036,
U.S.A.

British Library Cataloguing in Publication Data

Greene, John Gerald
 The social and psychological origins of the climacteric syndrome.
 1. Menopause
 I. Title
 612'.665   RG186

ISBN 0 566 00795 9

Typesetting by
MG Photoset, Pearce Lodge, University Avenue, Glasgow G12 8QQ
Printed and bound in Great Britain by
Biddles Ltd, Guildford and King's Lynn

Contents

List of Tables and Figures viii

Acknowledgements xii

Preface xiii

1
Menopause and Climacteric 1

    1.1. The Menopause   2
    1.2. The Climacteric   4
    1.3. Definition of Terms   8

2

Oestrogen and Climacteric Symptoms   12

    2.1. Symptoms of Oestrogen Deficiency: Clinical Opinions   13
    2.2. Oestrogen Replacement and Symptoms: Early Reports   15
    2.3. Oestrogen Replacement and Symptoms:
            Controlled Clinical Trials   18
    2.4. Psychotropic Effects of Oestrogen   31
    2.5. Summary and Conclusion   37

3

Symptoms During the Climacteric Among Women in the General Population   40

    3.1. Surveys of Symptoms   41
    3.2. Review of Surveys   44
    3.3. Summary and Conclusion   71

4

Other Aspects of Women's Functioning During the Climacteric   74

    4.1. The International Health Foundation Studies   75
    4.2. Sexual Functioning During the Climacteric   80
    4.3. Psychiatric Illness During the Climacteric   91
    4.4. Summary and Conclusion   98

5

Psychosocial Determinants of Women's Responses During the Climacteric   100

    5.1. Psychosocial Transition   101
    5.2. Studies of Psychosocial Transition   103
    5.3. Sociodemographic Factors   116
    5.4. Summary and Conclusion   131

6

Sociocultural Determinants of Women's Responses During the Climacteric — 134

    6.1. Studies of Attitudes to the Menopause — 135
    6.2. Cultural Variation — 146
    6.3. Summary and Conclusion — 160

7

Methodological Issues in Climacteric Research — 164

    7.1. General Considerations — 165
    7.2. Operational Definitions of Menopausal and Climacteric Status — 167
    7.3. The Assessment of Climacteric Symptoms — 170
    7.4. Factor Analytic Studies of Climacteric Symptoms — 174

8

Life Events During the Climacteric — 186

    8.1. Life Event Research — 187
    8.2. A Study of Life Events and Climacteric Symptoms — 190
    8.3. Discussion — 199

9

A Vulnerability Model of the Climacteric — 209

Bibliography — 220

Author Index — 238

Subject Index — 243

List of Tables and Figures

Tables

1.1.	Estimates of median age of menopause in seven different countries	4
1.2.	Example of a checklist of 'typical menopausal' symptoms	7
2.1.	Summary of controlled trials of the effect of oestrogen replacement on climacteric symptoms	19
2.2.	Symptoms improved by oestrogen therapy when compared with placebo	26
3.1.	Summary of the method of general population surveys of symptoms during the climacteric	43

3.2.	Average number of symptoms in relation to age and menopausal status	46
3.3.	Average number of symptoms in relation to menopausal status	54
3.4.	Comparison between clinical and general population groups on symptom scales	63
3.5.	Summary of the outcome of general population surveys of symptoms during the climacteric	69
3.6.	Prevalence of symptoms among menopausal women in five surveys	70
4.1.	Psychological and social characteristics examined in the International Health Foundation surveys	76
4.2.	Percentage of women complaining of loss of libido postoperatively	87
4.3.	The relation between sexual anxieties and postoperative sexual response	87
4.4.	Pre and posttreatment scores for three measures of sexual behaviour, vasomotor and psychological symptoms	90
4.5.	Percentages of depressed women having two of the DSMM criteria for involutional depression	95
5.1.	Summary of studies investigating effects of psychosocial factors on climacteric women	104
5.2.	Number of climacteric women with and without symptoms in relation to sex of marrying child	108
5.3.	Mean number of symptoms in relation to marital adjustment and child rearing stages	113
5.4.	Mean number of symptoms in relation to menopausal status and marital adjustment	114
5.5.	Median total symptom scores in relation to sociodemographic variables	117
5.6.	Percentage incidence of psychic and somatic symptoms in relation to socioeconomic status	120
5.7.	Percentage of women reporting symptoms in relation to educational attainment	122
5.8.	Sociodemographic factors and climacteric symptoms	130
6.1.	Summary of empirical studies of attitudes to the menopause	136
6.2.	Mean percentages of women agreeing to statements within each attitude category for each age group	138
6.3.	Percentages of positive responses in attitude towards the menopause	140

6.4. Attitude to the menopause of
Israeli women in relation to earlier psychosexual experience   145
6.5. Summary of cross cultural studies
of women's responses during the climacteric   148
6.6. Mean symptom scores of five ethnic groups in Israel   154
6.7. Mean number of symptoms reported by Navajo women   156
6.8. Percentages of women showing
negative responses for three attitude categories   158

7.1. Comparison of two methods of defining menopausal status   168
7.2. Rotated factor loadings of climacteric symptoms   177
7.3. Rotated factor loadings of climacteric symptoms   179
7.4. Symptoms with high loadings on each factor   181
7.5. A climacteric symptom rating scale   184

8.1. Significances of the relationships
between total life stress, menopausal status and symptoms   194
8.2. Mean total symptom
scores in relation to miscellaneous stress and deaths   198
8.3. Mean scores on the psychological and somatic symptom
scales in relation to miscellaneous stress and deaths   198

Figures

1.1. Potential sources of climacteric symptomatology   10

3.1. Examples of three types of symptom patterns:
per cent prevalance   48
3.2. Mean number of symptoms in relation to menopausal status   52
3.3. Cluster analysis of the relationship
between menopausal status and symptoms   53
3.4. Percentages of women with total climacteric index greater
than eleven points in relation to age and menopausal status   58
3.5. Mean scores for two symptom measures
in relation to menopausal status   60
3.6. Mean symptom scale scores in relation to climacteric status   62
3.7. Percentages of women reporting symptoms
in relation to menopausal status   64

4.1. Percentages of women showing good subjective adaptation
and good relations with spouse in relation to age
and menopausal status   77

4.2.	Percentages of women showing high independence and good normative integration in relation to age and menopausal status	78
4.3.	Percentages of women showing good subjective adaptation and normative integration in relation to menopausal status	79
4.4.	Percentages of women reporting sexual problems in relation to age	81
4.5.	Index of sexual pleasures in relation to age and menopausal status	82
4.6.	Sexual interest (per cent strong — moderate), capacity for orgasm (per cent always — occasionally) and frequency of coitus (number per year) in relation to age	84
5.1.	Percentages of women with climacteric index greater than eleven points in relation to menopausal status and maternal role	106
5.2.	Mean scores on two symptom scales in relation to social class	119
5.3.	Index of subjective adaptation in relation to social class	124
5.4.	Index of cultural activities in relation to social class	125
5.5.	Percentage of women reporting flushes in relation to employment and social class	126
5.6.	Mean scores on the nervosity index in relation to employment and social class	127
5.7.	Percentage of women showing good subjective adaptation in relation to employment and social class	128
8.1.	Mean scores for total life stress and its two main subcategories in relation to climacteric status	193
8.2.	Schematic diagram of the main categories of life stress during the climacteric	196
8.3.	Mean stress scores for two subcategories of exits in relation to climacteric status	196
8.4.	Schematic diagram of relationship between life events and climacteric symptoms in a sample of urban Scottish women, using Brown's terminology	207
9.	A vulnerability model of the climacteric	218

Acknowledgements

I wish to acknowledge the following authors, journals and publishers from whose works illustrative material has been adapted or reproduced. Numbers in parentheses refer to figures and tables in the present text.

G. Bungay et al. and *British Medical Journal* (Figure 4.4); C. Campagnoli et al. and *Maturitas* (Table 5.6); S. Campbell, M. Whitehead and W.D. Saunders and Company (Table 2.2); M. Crawford, D. Hooper and *Social Science and Medicine* (Table 5.2); D.L. Davis and the Memorial University of Newfoundland (Table 6.8); K. Dege, J. Gretzinger and the University of Texas Press (Table 6.3); L. Dennerstein et al. and *Obstetrics and Gynaecology* (Table 4.3); M. Dow et al. and *British Journal of Obstetrics and Gynaecology* (Table 4.4); T. Hallstrom and W.D. Saunders and Company (Figure 4.6); A. Holte, A. Mikkelsen and *Psychiatry and Social Science* (Table 7.4); B. Jaszmann et al. and *Medical Gynaecology and Sociology* (Figure 3.1, Table 5.5); P. Kaufert, J. Syrotuik and *Social Science and Medicine* (Table 7.3 and Figure 3.7); P. van Keep, H. Kellerhals and the International Health Foundation (Figures 3.4, 4.1, 4.2, 4.5, 5.1, 5.3, 5.4); S. McKinlay, M. Jefferys and *British Journal of Preventive and Social Medicine* (Figures 3.2, 3.3); B. Maoz et al. *Social Psychiatry* (Table 6.4) and *Acta Obstetrica Gynecologia Scandinavica* (Table 6.6); *Maturitas* (Figures 8.1, 8.3 and Tables 8.2, 8.3); B. Neugarten et al, and *Psychosomatic Medicine* (Table 1.2, 3.2) and *Vita Humana* (Table 6.2); L. Severne and MTP Press (Figures 3.5, 4.3, 5.5, 5.6, 5.7); C. Uphold, E. Susman and *Nursing Research* (Tables 5.3, 5.4); W. Utian and *International Journal of Gynaecology and Obstetrics* (Table 4.2); M.M. Weissman and *Journal of the American Medical Association* (Table 4.5); A.L. Wright and *Maturitas* (Table 6.7).

Preface

The last two decades have seen an upsurge of interest among medical and social scientists in the social and psychological aspects of the menopause and climacteric period of women's lives. This interest has generated a now substantial body of empirical research, which has been contributed to by various professional groups including nurses, sociologists, psychologists, psychiatrists, gynaecologists and anthropologists. The object of this book is firstly to present a comprehensive account of this work, which has appeared in diverse publications and which to the author's knowledge is not available elsewhere within a single volume, and secondly, on the basis of this account, to construct a cohesive sociopsychological model of the climacteric.

Throughout this book, the emphasis is on empirically based research; that is studies conforming to the methods of investigation developed over the years in the different behavioural sciences, in which the generation of empirical data is regarded as a first essential step. Within the behavioural sciences, data bases tend to be built up piece by piece from small scale circumscribed studies, rather than any one definitive large scale investigation. Nevertheless, knowledge derived in this way is not merely an accummulation of 'factual' material. Firstly, any general conclusions or interpretations must be based on a consideration of all research studies, some of which may conflict in their findings. Thus individual research findings must be evaluated against one another, in the process of which the quality of research design is of critical importance. Secondly, it must be recognised that data generated in the behavioural sciences is not entirely divorced from the methodology employed by the investigator. Nor is its interpretation divorced from the assumptions and perspectives the investigator or reviewer brings to the subject matter. The present author's background is that of a behavioural scientist whose applied experience is that of a clinician within a health service setting. It will be apparent that these influences have determined the selection and organisation of the material covered and the structural form this book has taken.

It will also be readily noted that the main dependent variable throughout is symptomatology. This not only conforms to the author's experience as a clinician, but it also reflects the vast bulk of medical and social science research in this field. The reason for this is that, for good or bad, 'illness behaviour' is one of the commonest ways individuals experience or express their reactions to adversity. The main focus is therefore on the concept of the 'climacteric syndrome', although whether such an entity has any validity depends, as is argued in the first chapter, on what the 'climacteric' is taken to refer to, and how rigorously the term 'syndrome' is used.

In the opening chapter, therefore, key terms are defined, and this determines how they will be used throughout the book. In the second chapter the relevant biomedical research is examined to see to what extend oestrogen deficiency contributes to the climacteric syndrome, particularly those symptoms and problems of a psychological nature. Chapters 3 to 6 contain an account of the existing sociopsychological research and this forms the core of the book. The first two of these chapters documents the changes — symptomatic, psychological and social — which take place among climacteric women, and in Chapters 5 and 6 possible factors contributing to these changes are examined. In Chapter 7 some problems of scientific method are discussed in relation to previous research and this leads in Chapter 8 to an account of the author's own research work on life events during the climacteric. The book concludes in Chapter 9 with an attempt to integrate these diverse findings into a cohesive and parsimonious sociopsychological model of the climacteric, based on the author's own research and that of others. This model, which is couched in terms of concepts developed in life event research, not only eschews a purely biomedical approach to the climacteric but it also questions some of the common assumptions regarding the 'social and psychological origins of the climacteric syndrome'.

I wish to take the opportunity to record my gratitude to Professor G.C. Timbury, Dean of Postgraduate Medicine, University of Glasgow, for his support and encouragement over the years. I am also indebted to Miss Carole Dempster, my personal secretary, who typed the initial drafts and to Miss June McKill, of the Lansdowne Clinic, who typed the final manuscript.

J.G. Greene
Glasgow, April 1984.

1

Menopause and Climacteric

At the outset, it is necessary to establish what precisely is meant by the climacteric and its associated terms. The purpose of this first chapter is to clarify the meaning of certain key terms in order to arrive at clear conceptual definitions, and this will determine the way they will be used throughout this volume. To do this it is necessary to begin with a brief account of the biological basis of the climacteric as many of these terms have their origins in the biomedical literature. This account is therefore confined to those aspects of biology relevant to that purpose. Those wishing to obtain a more detailed and comprehensive account of the biological and medical aspects of the climacteric should consult the excellent monograph by Utian (1980) — *Menopause in Modern Perspective: A Guide to Clinical Practice.*

1.1. THE MENOPAUSE

Some time in their middle years, women experience a final cessation of their menstrual cycle. This may occur abruptly or follow menstrual cycles of varying intervals with varying menstrual flow. This final cessation of periods, known as the menopause, is only one of the many consequences of a hormonal change which may well have been going on for some years, namely, dysfunction and failure of the ovaries.

Ovarian Failure

In the female reproductive system the ovaries contain oocytes. These are eggs at an immature stage, which develop into the follicles. These in turn erupt to produce the mature ovum capable of fertilisation by the male sperm. At birth the female ovary contains a finite number of oocytes of the order of some four hundred thousand (Block, 1952). No new eggs are produced in the woman's life time. The reason for ovarian failure is not clearly understood, but it is reasonable to suppose that at least one reason is that the ovary simply runs out of oocytes. By the time a woman is 45 to 50 years the number of oocytes is very low as a result of loss through ovulation and even more so through the process of atresia, that is the failure of several oocytes to mature to the follicular stage in each cycle. It is this depletion of the oocyte stock which ultimately leads to the menopause, loss of fertility, and the accompanying state of hormonal imbalance. This comes about in the following way.

The Reproductive Hormones

It is by the action of a stimulating or gonadotrophic hormone from the pituitary gland, follicle stimulating hormone (FSH), that the oocyte matures into a follicle. During this phase of the cycle the oocyte produces oestrogen, a hormone which has many target organs including the breasts, cervix, vagina and uterus. In the last organ, for example, it causes thickening of the lining or endometrium of the uterus, in preparation for implantation of a fertilised ovum. When the mature follicle erupts to shed the ovum, more oestrogen is produced along with another ovarian hormone progesterone, by the action of a second pituitary hormone, luteinising hormone (LH).

If no fertilised ovum is implanted these two ovarian hormones, oestrogen and progesterone, fall to a low level, the endometrium sheds, and menstruation occurs. In response to this fall, gonadotrophic hormones from the pituitary now start to rise again to initiate another cycle. The levels of ovarian and pituitary hormones are thus controlled by a feedback mechanism which ensures that as one falls the other rises. When, at the time of ovarian failure, the production of oestrogen cannot be maintained, partly because of depletion of the oocyte stock and partly because of the failure of those that remain to respond to gonadotrophin, this feedback mechanism results in a disproportionate increase in circulatory pituitary hormones. Around the time of the menopause, therefore, women enter a state of hormonal imbalance, as oestrogen levels fall and gonadotrophin hormones rise.

Age of Menopause

Despite variations in the method used for its estimation, the median age at which the menopause occurs has been found to be remarkably consistent across studies. Table 1.1 shows the range for studies carried out in seven countries to be from 50.0 to 51.5 years. It is clear then that the age of the menopause in these developed countries is around 50 years. The same cannot be said for third world countries. In a group of Punjabi women the median was found to be 44.0 years (Wyon et al., 1966) and Scragg (quoted in Gray, 1976) calculated the median to be 45.4 years in a group of women in New Guinea. It is thought that these differences may be due to the wide variations in health, nutrition and in general socioeconomic conditions which exist between developed and underdeveloped countries.

Although the age of menarche has fallen over the past century in developed countries (Tanner, 1962), also because of improved health and nutrition, the assumption that the age of menopause has increased for the same reasons is without foundation. Amundsen and Diers (1973) in a review of the medieval literature reported that in eight sources, from between the sixth and fifteenth century, 50 years was cited as the average age of menopause, and there is no evidence that this has changed over the last century (Gray, 1976).

The general consensus appears to be that the natural menopause occurs around a median age of 50 years in industrialised societies and that this has always been the case. Moreover, within developed countries it does not seem to be greatly affected by variations in socioeconomic conditions, race, marital status, income, geography or number of pregnancies (MacMahon and Worcester, 1966), although others have found some evidence that marital status and parity are related to age at menopause, independently of each other (McKinlay et al., 1972). For a fuller account of these and other issues associated with age at menopause see Gray (1976) or Brand (1978).

Table 1.1
Estimates of Median Age of Menopause in Seven Different Countries

Authors	Country	Median Age
MacMahon and Worcester (1966)	United States	50.0
Burch and Gunz (1967)	New Zealand	50.7
Jaszmann et al. (1969a)	Netherlands	51.4
Frere (1971)	South Africa	50.4
McKinlay et al. (1972)	England	50.8
Thompson et al. (1973)	Scotland	50.1
Brand (1978)	Netherlands	51.5

1.2. THE CLIMACTERIC

Unlike the menopause, which is a circumscribed and well defined event, ovarian failure is a gradual and prolonged process and is less easy to determine. The process of hormonal alteration to a new steady state has been estimated to take several years, with endocrine changes continuing beyond the actual cessation of menses (Sherman et al., 1976). It has been suggested by Studd et al. (1977a) that this may begin as long as ten years before the final cessation of menses and continue for some years thereafter. This prolonged period during which a woman experiences decreasing fertility, the menopause and the effects consequent on hormonal imbalance is known as the climacteric. This state of hormonal imbalance, and in particular the deficiency of oestrogen, is thought to give rise to a number of discomforting symptoms which women may experience at any time during the climacteric, but particularly around the time of the menopause.

Atrophic Vaginitis

One of the effects of oestrogen deficiency is to reduce secretions in the walls of the vagina. This leads to atrophy of the cells lining the vaginal walls and may cause vaginal dryness and irritation, vaginitis and on occasion pain on intercourse (dyspareunia). These are the symptoms of atrophic vaginitis, and they are among the earliest of climacteric symptoms to occur (Utian, 1980, Chapter 7).

Vasomotor Symptoms

Perhaps the most common and best known of symptoms associated with the menopause and the climacteric are hot flushes. These are usually described as a sudden sensation of heat rising from the chest to the neck and face, together with diffuse or patchy flushing of the skin. This vasodilation is followed by vasoconstriction, so that after a flush may come a cold shiver. Flushes may also be accompanied by bouts of sweating, often occurring at night. These irregularities and extremes of bodily temperature are collectively known as vasomotor symptoms, and they too are among the earliest and most characteristic of climacteric symptoms. It is generally considered that like atrophic vaginitis they too come about as a result of hormonal imbalance, although the actual mechanism of vasomotor symptoms has still to be elucidated. They cannot be explained by low oestrogen levels alone nor solely by elevated gonadotrophin, as extreme levels of either may occur in other conditions without producing vasomotor instability (Studd et al., 1977a).

Furthermore, no association has as yet been found between the presence of vasomotor symptoms and levels of ovarian or pituitary hormones. For example, Aksel et al. (1976) found no statistically significant differences in total serum oestrogen, FSH and LH concentrations between groups of patients with and without vasomotor symptoms, following removal of the ovaries (oophorectomy). Similar failures to find any relationship between plasma levels of ovarian and pituitary hormones and the occurrence of vasomotor symptoms have been reported by Hunter et al. (1973), Stone et al. (1975), Chakravarti et al. (1977) and Dennerstein et al. (1978). Hutton et al. (1978), although finding dyspareunia (a symptom of atrophic vaginitis) to be associated with low plasma-oestradiol concentrations in a mixed group of natural menopausal and oophorectomised women, found no relation between hot flushes and particular concentrations, mean levels or pattern of fluctuation of plasma-oestrone or oestradiol. These last authors suggest that as there is no clear relation between onset of flushes and oestrogen levels, a more complex relation, such as changes in autonomic activity by alteration in levels of oestrogen metabolites in the central nervous system, may be involved. Another possibility, suggested by Utian (1980, Chapter 7), is that it is the rate of decline, rather than absolute levels of oestrogen concentration that is responsible. Despite their ubiquity the precise aetiology of vasomotor symptoms remains obscure.

Later Symptoms

These early manifestations of oestrogen deficiency — symptoms of atrophic vaginitis and vasomotor instability — are often distinguished from the later effects. As all tissues of the body may, to some extent, be regarded as target organs for oestrogen, the entire organism may therefore suffer from increasing oestrogen deficiency. It has been suggested that not all tissues react at the same time and for this reason later symptoms may follow a temporal sequence with skin atrophy being followed by osteoporosis, being followed by atherosclerosis (van Keep and Kellerhals, 1973). In view of the fact that the menopause occurs at a time of life when there is a rising incidence of degenerative disease, it is not surprising that causal relationships between some of these degenerative disorders and endocrine change should have been postulated. However, evidence for these relationships tends to be of an indirect nature (see Utian, 1980, Chapter 4).

The 'Menopausal Syndrome'

Despite an incomplete understanding of the actual mechanism whereby oestrogen deficiency results in vasomotor instability, the characteristic occurrence of these symptoms, together with a number of others around the time of the menopause, has given rise to the notion of a 'menopausal syndrome'. In medical parlance a symptom is defined as a subjective phenomenon or manifestation of a disease. Syndrome refers to a group of symptoms and/or signs which occurring together produce a symptom pattern typical of a particular disease or medical condition.

Many middle aged women coming to hospital clinics and general practitioners' surgeries complaining of vasomotor symptoms and atrophic vaginitis in association with menstrual irregularity or cessation, also complain of a variety of other distressing symptoms. These symptoms are diverse and range from what seem physical symptoms, such as rheumatic pains, dizzy spells, numbness and tingling of extremities, palpitations, breathlessness, cold hands and feet, to what seem to be symptoms of psychological distress — irritability, anxiety, crying spells, depression and so forth. It is to this constellation of symptoms that the term 'menopausal syndrome' is commonly applied.

Table 1.2
Example of a Checklist of 'Typical Menopausal' Symptoms

Somatic	Psychosomatic	Psychological
Hot flushes	Tired feelings	Irritable and nervous
Cold Sweats	Headaches	Feeling blue and depressed
Weight gain	Pounding of heart	Forgetfulness
Flooding	Dizzy spells	Excitable
Rheumatic pains	Blind spots before the eyes	Trouble sleeping
Aches in back of neck and skull		Cannot concentrate
Cold hands and feet		Crying spells
Numbness and tingling		Feelings of suffocation
Breast pains		Worry about body
Constipation		Feelings of fright or panic
Diarrhoea		Worry about nervous breakdown
Skin crawls		

Adapted from Neugarten and Kraines (1965)

In practice, unfortunately, the term is used loosely and in an overinclusive way, in that almost any non-specific distress or discomfort experienced by women in middle life, may be attributed to the 'menopausal syndrome', thereby implying that the menopause has some sort of aetiological significance for such complaints. By non-specific in this context is meant any complaints or symptoms which cannot be accounted for by a known medical or psychiatric condition. Table 1.2 shows a typical example of a list of this sort, in which symptoms are itemised in what Utian (1980) refers to as the 'grocery list style' (p.106). In a review of the medical literature on the menopause, the present author (Greene, 1976) arrived at a list of no less than 45 different symptoms of this sort, all of which had been attributed to the menopause by some author at some time. Indeed, in clinical practice, the term 'menopausal syndrome' is sometimes applied to middle aged women complaining of such non-specific and diverse symptoms, not only in the absence of symptoms of vasomotor instability or atrophic vaginitis, but also in the absence of any sign of menstrual irregularity. The term is therefore a much abused one, and the aetiological contribution of the cessation of menses alone to such a plethora of symptoms must de facto be open to question. As shall be seen in the next section a more acceptable term for this constellation of symptoms might be 'climacteric syndrome'.

1.3. DEFINITION OF TERMS

It has frequently been suggested that much of the confusion in this field derives from a lack of clear and consistent definitions of basic terms such as menopause, climacteric, menopausal syndrome, climacteric syndrome and oestrogen deficiency syndrome.

Consensus on Definitions

A useful starting point is the report of a Workshop convened during the First International Congress on the Menopause, held at La Grande Motte in France in 1976. The task of this Workshop was to arrive at an agreed set of definitions for some of the key terms used in climacteric research. In their report on this Workshop, Utian and Serr (1976) proposed the following definitions:

1. The climacteric was defined as that phase in the ageing process of women marking the transition from the reproductive stage of life to the non-reproductive stage.
2. The menopause referred to the final menstrual period and occurs during the climacteric.

3. The climacteric is sometimes, but not necessarily always, associated with symptomatology. When this does occur it may be termed the 'climacteric syndrome'.

Climacteric symptoms and complaints were regarded as being derived from three main sources:

1. Decreased ovarian activity with subsequent hormonal deficiency, resulting in early symptoms (hot flushes, perspiration and atrophic vaginitis) and late symptoms related to metabolic changes in the end organ affected.
2. Sociocultural factors determined by the woman's environment.
3. Psychological factors, dependent on the woman's character.

The variety of symptomatology was seen to be the result of interaction between these three sources.

A number of important points arise from the foregoing definitions. The term climacteric is being used in a developmental sense to cover a transitional phase in the life span during which a woman moves from being reproductive to being non-reproductive. This can occur over a lengthy period of time and includes not merely the process of physical ageing, hormonal changes and the menopause itself, but also any psychological or social changes contingent on this transition.

The absence of a menopausal *syndrome* should be noted. This seems to imply that there is no syndrome as such contingent on the event of the menopause. This is made more explicit by van Keep (1979) in editorial advice to prospective authors regarding the use of terminology in the then newly founded journal *Maturitas*. This advice was based on guidelines issued by the Nomenclature Committee of the International Federation of Gynaecology and Obstetrics. Van Keep advises authors to note the following definitions:

> The climacteric is the phase in the ageing process during which a woman passes from the reproductive to the non-reproductive stage. The signals that this period of life has been reached are to be referred to as climacteric symptoms or, if more serious as climacteric complaints (not as menopausal symptomatology nor menopausal complaints). The menopause is the final menstruation which occurs during the climacteric (p.227).

The consensus is that the menopause is merely an event occurring within the climacteric, being one of the consequences of oestrogen deficiency. It is therefore a *sign* of oestrogen deficiency or, more correctly, a sign that a critical point has been reached in the oestrogen deficiency process. The question which many writers ask, as to what are the symptoms of the menopause does not arise. A more appropriate question would be — what are the symptoms of oestrogen deficiency? This does not of course exclude the possibility of the menopause exercising some specific influences of its own, either physical or psychological, or even of a symbolic nature, as part of the total climacteric picture, but not constituting a separate syndrome.

The Climacteric Syndrome

The term 'climacteric syndrome', however, is used, and any symptoms and complaints thought to be associated in any way with a woman's transition from being reproductive to non-reproductive, would logically be seen as part of this syndrome. Therefore, although the climacteric is defined in terms of a change in biological function, namely reproductive capacity, the symptoms of the climacteric are not necessarily of biological origin. They could have a variety of origins. Some might be directly due to oestrogen deficiency, some might be a response to the menopause itself, some a result of the general effects of ageing and still others a function of psychological and sociocultural factors related, directly or otherwise, to the menopause or climacteric. These sources are schematically illustrated in Figure 1.1. This entails a departure from the strict medical use of the terms symptom and syndrome, as defined in the preceding section. It

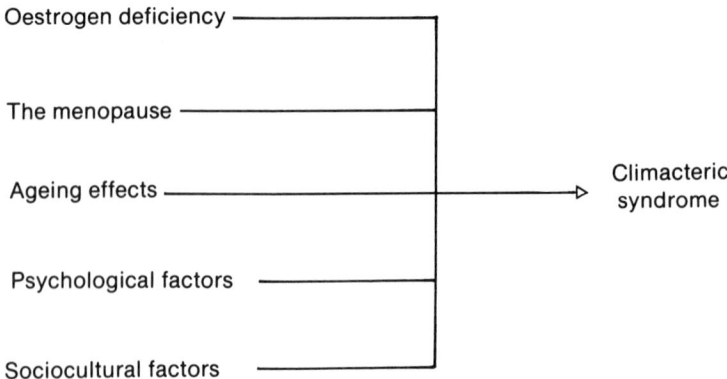

Figure 1.1 Potential sources of climacteric symptomatology.

constitutes a much looser use of both terms, in which symptoms are taken not so much as manifestations of a circumscribed disease but more an expression of *dis*-ease of multiple origins, and in which the term syndrome is confined not purely to symptoms but may include other complaints and adverse effects.

The question still remains, however, as to which symptoms and complaints are part of the overall climacteric syndrome and of these, which are a function of the menopause itself, and which are derived from the three main sources of climacteric symptoms, namely, decreased ovarian activity, sociocultural factors and psychological factors. The answers to these questions are of course open to empirical investigation and are the subject matter of the remainder of this volume.

2

Oestrogen and Climacteric Symptoms

We have seen in Chapter 1 the central role played by decreased ovarian activity and declining oestrogen levels in bringing about the menopause, infertility and other physical changes during the climacteric. The question we now address ourselves to is — of all the symptoms making up the climacteric syndrome, which can be confidently attributed to oestrogen deficiency? In this chapter the role of oestrogen in the aetiology of the climacteric syndrome, and in particular those symptoms of a psychological nature, is examined. In doing this we begin by presenting current medical opinion on this issue, in order to illustrate the diversity of views on this matter, before moving onto a review of the therapeutic effects of oestrogen replacement therapy. This review is based on an analysis of recent controlled trials of the effects of oestrogen replacement on climacteric symptoms, especially the psychological ones, and it forms the centre piece of the chapter.

2.1. SYMPTOMS OF OESTROGEN DEFICIENCY: CLINICAL OPINIONS

There is a general consensus among clinicians and researchers that symptoms of vasomotor instability and those of atrophic vaginitis are among the earliest and most characteristic of symptoms of the climacteric. There is also general agreement that these symptoms are in some way a consequence of oestrogen deficiency (Utian, 1980, Chapter 4). Nor is there much doubt that, among women presenting at clinics and surgeries, these symptoms are frequently accompanied by a variety of non-specific physical and psychological symptoms, such as those described in section 1.2. Opinions have varied, however, as to the nature of the relationship between vasomotor symptoms and these other physical and psychological symptoms, and the role played by oestrogen deficiency in the aetiology of such symptoms.

Two opposing viewpoints can be identified here. The conservative position has been to regard only vasomotor symptoms and those of atrophic vaginitis as being directly due to oestrogen deficiency. Here are two examples of this viewpoint:

> There was a general feeling that hot flushes, perspiration, atrophic vaginitis, are the only true early features of lack of oestrogen and that a different explanation must be sought to account for all the other symptoms usually attributed to oestrogen deficiency or listed as part of the climacteric syndrome. (Utian and Serr, 1976, p.2)

> In fact there are only two typical climacteric complaints; hot flushes and bouts of perspiration. Both seem directly related to the sudden decrease of the production of estrogenic hormone. There are a whole series of other symptoms which are sometimes regarded as being part of the climacteric picture. Most of these are not very specific and may also occur in other phases of life. (Haspels and van Keep, 1979, p.61)

A dissenting voice, even from this conservative position is that of Mulley and Mitchell (1976), who writing in *The Lancet* conclude:

> Thus, no correlation has so far been established between hormonal changes and menopausal flushing .... we contend that there is no clear-cut relation between hot flushes and oestrogen deficiency. (p.1398).

At the other extreme however, some writers seem to imply that not only are vasomotor symptoms caused directly by oestrogen deficiency but that many of the other physical and psychological symptoms are also so caused. That is, they too have a *direct* hormonal basis. For example:

> The menopause is often accompanied by a number of physical and a great variety of disturbing psychological alterations which in fact, appear well in advance, in the premenopausal period. As they correlate fairly well with the diminishing oestrogen level, most of them are thought to be the consequence of progressive oestrogen deficiency. (Kopera, 1973, p.124)

> The menopause is often accompanied by a great variety of disturbing psychological alterations which often arise in the pre-menopausal period and correlate fairly well with the diminishing oestrogen level. (Oram and Chakravarti, 1975, p.16)

> Psychological changes of anxiety, depression, tension and irritability apparently begin long before the actual termination of periods and correlate fairly well with oestrogen levels. (Kerr, 1976, p.27)

Between these two opposing positions are a range of modifications of them. In some of these modifications at least some of the other symptoms are thought to be directly due to oestrogen deficiency. In others, although other symptoms are not seen as being directly caused by oestrogen deficiency, it is thought that the deficiency may serve to exacerbate such symptoms, if they are already present for other reasons. Alternatively, it may be considered that although some of the other symptoms are directly caused by oestrogen deficiency, they may be exacerbated by other factors, psychological or social. Finally, while it may be agreed that only vasomotor symptoms are directly caused by oestrogen deficiency, it is considered that the discomfort of these unpleasant symptoms may give rise to other complaints. Within each of these positions there are differences of opinion as to which particular symptoms are involved. Here are three examples of these varying positions:

> The emotional changes (during the climacteric) are of multi factorial etiology, and the climacteric may only accentuate a pre-existing psychic insufficiency. (Bodnar and Catterill, 1972, p.3)

> The climacteric uncloaks many of the neurotic and psychogenic symptoms that women have managed to suppress until then. (Lauritzen, 1973, p.5)

> Patients who suffered from hot flushes more often complained of headache, dyspareunia, pains in muscles and joints and insomnia, possibly due to night sweats. These complaints may be regarded as related to the climacteric. (Chakravarti et al., 1979, p.985)

It is clear from the foregoing, therefore, that there is considerable disagreement in the medical literature as to what are the 'true' symptoms of oestrogen deficiency, and this final quotation from Studd et al. (1977a) is probably a fair summary of current medical opinion on this issue:

> There is a lack of general agreement as to the precise symptomatology of the climacteric and, in particular, it can be most difficult to separate the valid symptoms of oestrogen deficiency from symptoms of ageing and the effects of social and domestic problems of the middle-aged woman. (p.8)

2.2. OESTROGEN REPLACEMENT AND SYMPTOMS: EARLY REPORTS

It might be thought that a definitive way of resolving the question as to which symptoms are due to oestrogen deficiency might be by determining which of the many symptoms attributed to the menopause respond to oestrogen therapy. Such treatment has been available now for almost half a century. Modern oestrogen treatment has its origins in the discovery by Butenandt and others in 1929 of oestrone, the first biologically active steroid to be isolated (Utian, 1980, Chapter 1). From then it was but a small step to the development of oestrogenic preparations in biologically assayed forms as medication for the clinical management of patients. The logic of administering oestrogen to menopausal women is clearly to make up for the oestrogen loss occurring at that time, and by doing so to relieve those symptoms thought to be directly due to a deficiency of this hormone.

From the beginning claims were made that oestrogen therapy not only relieved the characteristic hot flushes and sweats, but that it also alleviated the variety of other somatic and psychological complaints women experienced around that time. In effect the claim was made that the entire 'menopausal symptom complex' could be relieved by oestrogen therapy. To begin with these views were based either on personal clinical experience in prescribing oestrogen, or on published reports of the outcome of oestrogen therapy with series of patients attending gynaecological clinics.

Typical examples of the latter are the early papers by Sevringhaus (1935), Wiesbader and Kurzrok (1938) and Hawkinson (1938). These reports, emerging a few years after the development of the first dependable oestrogen based preparations, contained remarkable claims regarding their efficacy. The results in the series by Sevringhaus (1935) were so impressive that he concluded 'failure to obtain relief from the majority of subjective symptoms in uncomplicated menopause is usually due to inadequate dosage' (p.626). No figures, however, are published in this report. Hawkinson (1938) did report some crude figures, finding that in a series of 1000 women gathered over a six year period, 70 per cent were relieved of the majority of all symptoms and only 5 per cent experienced no relief of symptoms.

Around the same time, however, Pratt and Thomas (1937) were already initiating controversy about oestrogen by reporting that menopausal symptoms showed a substantial response to placebo, that is, inert preparations with no active pharmacological ingredients. In a double blind study, that is where neither doctor nor patient knew which preparations were being taken, these authors compared the efficacy of a number of oestrogen preparations with preparations containing plain oil and lactose. They found that 'regardless of the form of therapy the majority of patients are relieved or improved. Furthermore, there is only a slight difference indicated for the different agents used' (p.1877). The necessity for the use of a placebo in any study investigating the effect of oestrogen on climacteric symptoms had been demonstrated.

The most convincing and influential studies therefore proved to be those carried out in the fifties, in which oestrogen based preparations were compared with placebo, and on occasion other active preparations, such as phenobarbitol and Vitamin E, in large groups of women. Notable among these studies were those by Greenblatt et al. (1950), Kupperman et al. (1953) and Blatt et al. (1953). In the largest of these, that by Kupperman et al. (1953), 18 preparations were compared among a sample of 1400 women attending a gynaecological clinic over a period of several years using a double blind administration. Some 33 per cent of women showed a moderate to excellent response to placebo. This compared with a similar type of response in 92 per cent of women for the most effective oestrogen preparation (ethinyloestradiol) and 60 per cent for the least effective (stilbestrol). Similar results were obtained in the other two studies referenced above and also in a later and even larger scale study by Kupperman et al. (1959).

Nevertheless, despite the improved sophistication of design, these studies were still essentially clinical reports and not properly controlled trials in the modern sense. Furthermore, they threw no light on the differential responses of individual symptoms to oestrogen therapy since the outcome measures were fairly crude ones. For example, in the two reports by Kupperman et al. (1953, 1959), although a Menopausal Index containing eleven different symptoms was used to assess individual symptoms, outcome was based on 'consideration of both the menopausal index and clinical improvement'. In effect a global assessment of improvement was made of the patient's overall wellbeing, in which the alleviation of hot flushes appears to be the symptom most attended to. However, the implication in most of these reports was that the patient's general physical and psychological health had improved as a *direct* result of oestrogen therapy, and this came to be the generally accepted view. Oestrogen therapy consequently gained the reputation of being a panacea for all ills and complaints experienced by women in middle life. Others went further and saw it as a means of slowing down the ageing process in general. This position is well illustrated in the writings of the American physician, Robert Wilson whose views are aptly summarised in the title of his influential and best selling book, *Feminine Forever* (Wilson, 1966), and in other articles for example, Wilson and Wilson (1963). Wilson took the view that the postmenopause should be regarded as a period of pathological oestrogen deficiency which lasts from menopause until death, arguing persuasively that the administration of oestrogen in this phase of life could slow down a number of the phenomena of ageing. This somewhat doubtful assertion, although gaining wide acceptance in the media and among the population at large, was supported, in the words of Haspels and van Keep (1979), 'by combining the scanty clinical evidence available, with data from animal experiments and statements from grateful patients' (p.58).

Properly controlled trials of oestrogen replacement therapy did not in fact appear until the 1970s. By 'properly controlled trial' the present author means trials set up prospectively (not retrospective examination of case records) and which fulfil the following criteria:

1. An acceptable placebo procedure is used.
2. An attempt is made to render the trial at least single, but preferably double blind.
3. Outcome is assessed in a reasonably objective way, and different measures of outcome are employed. Outcome should therefore not be based merely on clinical judgement, and if possible existing standardised scales should be used.
4. In the analysis of the results there should be appropriate use of inferential statistics to ensure that differences between groups on outcome measures could not have arisen by chance.

These are the sort of design criteria which are now generally accepted as essential in order to demonstrate the efficacy or otherwise of active pharmacological preparations. Trials, fulfilling these criteria, of oestrogen preparations are now reviewed in the following section.

2.3. OESTROGEN REPLACEMENT AND SYMPTOMS: CONTROLLED CLINICAL TRIALS

The clinical trials to be reviewed in this section not only fulfil, for the most part, the criteria listed at the end of the previous section, they also have included in the outcome measures, an assessment of symptoms other than those due to vasomotor instability, in particular psychological ones. They are all therefore of relevance to the issue as to which of the many symptoms experienced by climacteric women are alleviated by oestrogen replacement. These trials are listed in Table 2.1 in which details of method and outcome of each trial are summarised. The trials are listed in the order in which they will be discussed. From time to time in the course of this review, references will be made to other trials of an uncontrolled nature, where it is thought that their findings are of some relevance to the discussion.

The trials listed in Table 2.1 are, with one exception (Utian, 1972a), all double blind, and are either of the simple randomised or crossover design. In both types of design subjects are allocated randomly either to a drug or placebo group, but whereas in the former design they remain on the same regime throughout the trial, in the latter case they are alternated at some point so that all subjects receive both placebo and oestrogen for a time. This should not be regarded as an exhaustive list of all published oestrogen trials. It includes only those in which an assessment of psychological symptoms has been carried out, and in which a placebo control has been used. The reason for this stricture is that of all symptoms, psychological ones are most notoriously subject to placebo effects.

Martin, Burnier, Segre and Huix (1971)

One of the first well designed modern trials of oestrogen therapy was that carried out by Martin et al. (1971). These authors compared a high and a low dose oestrogen preparation (ethinyloestradiol) with a placebo over a three month period in a double blind controlled trial. Daily flush count was recorded and ten other symptoms assessed. Both drug dosages resulted in a significant reduction in hot flushes over the trial period but were not significantly different in effect from each other. The placebo had no effect on hot flushes. With regard to other symptoms a decrease in one symptom only, 'nervousness', was observed with the two active drug preparations, but not the placebo group. Headaches improved equally in

Table 2.1

Summary of Controlled Trials of the Effect of Oestrogen Replacement on Climacteric Symptoms

Authors	Design and Time on Oestrogen (in weeks)	Oestrogen Preparation	Placebo Effect	Symptom Measures	Measure for which Effect of Oestrogen Greater than Placebo
Martin et al. (1971)	Randomised 12	Ethinyloestradiol	None	Daily flush count, 10 other symptoms	Hot flushes, nervousness
Jarvinen et al. (1971)	Randomised 24	Oestriol succinate	Large	Kupperman Index (12 symptoms)	Dyspareunia only
Aylward (1973)	Randomised 12	Piperazine oestrone	Not reported	Hamilton depression scale	Depression (but see text)
Thomson and Oswald (1977)	Randomised 8	Piperazine oestrone	Large	Weekly flush count, Hamilton scales, objective sleep measures	Sleep measures only
Utian (1972a, b)	Single blind sequential	Oestradiol valerate, conjugated equine	Moderate	14 symptoms, general wellbeing	Hot flushes, atrophic vaginitis, general wellbeing
George et al. (1973)	Crossover 4	Conjugated equine	Not reported	Minor psychiatric symptoms, Beck depression inventory	Hot flushes only
Strickler et al. (1977)	Crossover 12	Conjugated equine	Large	Overall wellbeing, 2 symptoms	None
Coope et al. (1975)	Crossover 12	Conjugated equine	Large	Weekly flush count, Kupperman index	Flushes (but see text)
Fedor-Freybergh (1977)	Randomised 12	Oestradiol valerate	None	Hamilton depression scale, symptom and distress scales	All three measures (vasomotor not reported)
Campbell and Whitehead (1977)	Crossover 8 and 24	Conjugated equine	Moderate	24 symptoms, Beck depression inventory, GHQ	See Table 2.2
Dennerstein et al. (1978; 1979)	Crossover 12	Ethinyloestradiol	Moderate	Flush count, 6 symptoms, Hamilton depression scale	Hot flushes, insomnia, Hamilton anxiety items
Schiff et al. (1979)	Crossover 4	Conjugated equine	Not reported	10 symptoms, objective sleep measures	Flushes, sleep measures
Paterson (1982)	Crossover 12	Ethinyloestradiol	Small	Weekly flush count, 23 symptoms	Flushes, sweating, insomnia
Nordin et al. (1980)	Randomised 3	Ethinyloestradiol	Small	18 symptom scale	Flushes mainly (individual symptoms not reported)
Ikeda et al. (1978)	Randomised 3	Conjugated equine	Large	Physician and patients overall rating	Neither rating (individual symptoms not reported)

both the high oestrogen and placebo groups, and breast pain became worse with the high oestrogen regimen. No significant changes were noted in any other symptoms, namely, depression, fatigue, insomnia, joint pains, leg aches, bloating and fluid retention for any of the three treatment groups. The two points to be noted from this study are the limited placebo effect on symptoms and the general absence of any improvement in non-vasomotor symptoms as a result of oestrogen therapy.

Jarvinen, Kokkenen and Rhyanen (1971)

The foregoing study stands in contrast on both these counts to another study reported around the same time by Jarvinen et al. (1971). In this double blind controlled trial, oestriol succinate was compared with a placebo, using as a measure of symptoms the Kuppermann Index (Kupperman et al., 1953). In this scale 12 symptoms were rated in terms of severity. These were hot flushes, sweating, paraesthesia, insomnia, nervousness, melancholia, vertigo, fatigue, arthralgia, headaches, palpitations and formication. It was found that both drug and placebo had an equal effect on all these symptoms with the exception of dyspareunia, which responded better to oestrogen. Unlike the study by Martin and his colleagues there was therefore a substantial placebo effect, which was equal to that of the active preparation.

Aylward (1973)

In contrast to both these studies, Aylward (1973), in a trial of piperazine oestrone sulphate claimed that this oestrogen preparation had a direct effect on depressive symptoms. Ten women received the active preparation and eight the placebo in a double blind administration over a three month period. Outcome was assessed by means of a standardised psychiatric scale, the Hamilton Depression Rating Scale (Hamilton, 1960). Unfortunately, for reasons best known to the author, no data were provided regarding actual changes in the depression ratings for either group. The claim that oestrogen had a beneficial effect on depression was based on a correlation between ranked changes in depressive ratings and plasma free tryptophan levels, a compound thought to be implicated in psychiatric depression (Coppen et al., 1973). Why pre and post trial mean scores for both placebo and drug groups were not reported for the Hamilton Scale is not at all clear.

Aylward et al. (1974), in a second trial comparing two oestrogen preparations, piperazine oestrone sulphate with that used by Martin et al. (1971), ethinyloestradiol, again obtained quite different results from the latter. This was a double blind crossover trial, with half the patients commencing on one drug and changing to the other after three weeks. There was a significant decrease in the frequency of vasomotor symptoms for both drugs, piperazine oestrone sulphate being the more effective. Both preparations also reduced insomnia, anxiety and depression, the last two being measured again by the Hamilton Rating Scales (Hamilton, 1959 and 1960). Unfortunately, although all patients received a placebo over the three weeks before commencing the active drugs, no comparisons were reported between drug and placebo effects. Placebo effects cannot therefore be evaluated. Furthermore, prior to commencing drug treatment 'placebo responders' were excluded from the trial. There were again certain peculiarities in the manner in which the psychological outcome measures were analysed in this study. All this makes these studies difficult ones to evaluate, and the authors' conclusions that oestrogen has a clear positive effect on the psyche appears premature. Certainly in this respect the findings of this research group stand out from all others.

Thomson and Oswald (1977)

Aylward's findings, for example, contrast markedly with those of Thomson and Oswald (1977) in a later well designed double blind trial in which the more effective of these drugs, piperazine oestrone sulphate, was compared, this time, with a placebo. Using exactly the same measures of anxiety and depression (the Hamilton Rating Scales) and a more orthodox method to quantify outcome, these authors found that mean scores on both scales improved steadily in both groups throughout the study, there being no difference between drug and placebo at any assessment point. A similar pattern was found in the case of hot flushes. The authors did find that the oestrogen preparation was, however, more effective in alleviating insomnia assessed by objective methods in a sleep laboratory. Thus, in this more convincing trial, the effect of this particular drug on almost all symptoms was indistinguishable from the large placebo effect.
    Of relevance here is a study by Coppen and Wood (1978) who, in a double blind crossover trial of conjugated oestrogen with a group of depressed female patients attending a psychiatric clinic, found that although there was an increase in the level of free tryptophan in response

to oestrogen there was no corresponding improvement in affective morbidity among these women as rated by a psychiatrist, nor was there on a standard rating scale, the Beck Depression Inventory (Beck et al., 1961). The relationship between tryptophan and depression however is a controversial one. Peet et al. (1976), for example, in a carefully controlled study found no significant changes in plasma total or free tryptophan levels in patients recovered from depressive psychosis. The reports of Aylward and his colleagues regarding the beneficial effect of oestrogen on depression must therefore be reconsidered in the light of these and later studies.

Also relevant to the finding of Thomson and Oswald (1977) regarding the beneficial effect of oestrogen on sleep is an earlier uncontrolled trial by Lozman et al. (1971). No placebo was used in this trial, piperazine oestrone sulphate being compared wth conjugated equine oestrogen, using a double blind crossover method. Both drugs were equally effective in reducing all symptoms — flushes, sweats, depression and anxiety — with the exception of insomnia which responded better to piperazine oestrone sulphate. This particular preparation might therefore have a specific sedative effect.

Utian (1972a,b)

Utian (1972a) in an earlier trial had also compared conjugated oestrogen with another oestrogen preparation, oestradiol valerate, this time in a placebo controlled trial. Subjects, all oophorectomised women, first received oestradiol valerate for six months, followed by the placebo for three months and then the conjugated oestrogen for a further three months. The study was therefore only single blind as the researcher knew which drug each patient was taking. In all 14 symptoms were assessed.

There was a significant improvement in hot flushes while women were on oestrogen, there being no differences in the effects of either drug. During the placebo phase hot flushes returned, but not entirely back to their original level. The symptoms of atrophic vaginitis followed a similar pattern. For five other symptoms, however, palpitations, insomnia, irritability, depression and angina pectoris, any relief while taking oestrogen was no greater than that during placebo. Three other symptoms, headaches, low backache and loss of libido, showed response to neither drug nor placebo. In this study therefore, there was a placebo effect on most symptoms, but only in the case of hot flushes and atrophic vaginitis was the effect of oestrogen significantly greater.

In a later paper Utian (1972b) did claim that there was evidence in this trial of a direct psychic effect from oestrogen, which he described as a 'mental tonic' effect. This was measured by means of a five point rating of the patient's general wellbeing based on the author's 'impression' of the patient in interview. During both oestrogen treatments this increased but declined during placebo. However, as the author knew which preparation the patient was taking the possibility of rater bias exists. Furthermore, even if there was a genuine improvement in the mental wellbeing of the patient there is no reason for supposing a direct hormonal effect on psychic functions, which seems to be the implication. What could be happening is that the relief from hot flushes and atrophic vaginitis produces the sense of wellbeing. This is an issue which will be returned to later in this review.

George, Utian, Beaumont and Beardwood (1973)

George et al. (1973), in another trial of conjugated oestrogen against placebo, set out specifically with the object of investigating the effect of oestrogen on what they call 'minor psychiatric symptoms', this time using a double blind crossover design. What these symptoms were, is not revealed, but they were assessed by means of a checklist, each symptom being rated in severity. The Beck Depression Inventory, a standardised measure of pyschiatric depression was also included. All patients reported relief of hot flushes when on oestrogen, followed by relapse when on placebo. No significant differences were found between oestrogen and placebo for the total score on the psychiatric symptoms measure, nor the Beck Index at the end of each treatment period. These authors conclude that their findings contrast with those reported by Utian (1972b) regarding the 'mental tonic' effect of oestrogen. However, it must be pointed out that Utian did not measure the 'mental tonic' effect in terms of the alleviation of individual symptoms, but did so in terms of his overall impression of the patient's wellbeing (see above). Indeed, the findings of George and his colleagues in respect to individual psychological symptoms, concur entirely with those of Utian, who found that for most of these the oestrogen effect was no greater than that of the placebo. Unfortunately, as no pretreatment scores were recorded in this trial, it is not possible to determine if there was a placebo effect.

Strickler and Colleagues (1977)

Relevant to this point are the results of a trial by Strickler et al. (1977) in which conjugated oestrogen was again compared with placebo. In this case the trial was again double blind with a crossover design. Although the principle focus of attention was on changes in personality consequent to oestrogen therapy, a measure based on a physician's interpretation of a woman's overall sense of wellbeing, not dissimilar to that used by Utian, was employed. An equal number of women, 17 out of 20 in each case, reported improvement on this measure regardless of what treatment they were receiving. In this case, of course, the study being double blind, the interviewer had no knowledge of what preparation the patient was receiving. As hot flushes also improved equally in response to both drug and placebo, the most likely conclusion is that the reported improvement in overall wellbeing was also due to a placebo effect or to the alleviation of vasomotor symptoms. It should be noted however, that as in the Utian study more specific symptoms, such as mood and energy level, showed little changes during either the oestrogen or placebo phases nor did scores on tests of personality. Once again, therefore, the effect of oestrogen on most symptoms was undistinguishable from the effects of the placebo.

Coope, Thomson and Poller (1975)

The potency of the placebo response was again illustrated in a double blind crossover trial of conjugated oestrogen against placebo over a six month period by Coope et al. (1975). Symptoms were assessed by means of the Kupperman Index (see Jarvinen et al. above) and a weekly hot flush count. In the first three months, that is prior to crossover, the total menopausal index score was greatly reduced by both placebo and oestrogen but the difference between them was not significant. During the second three month period women now taking oestrogen continued to improve, but those now on placebo worsened. Hot flush count followed the same pattern, only moreso. Thus there was a massive placebo response in the first but not second half of the trial. The authors account for the absence of a placebo response in the second part of the trial in terms of the changes in hot flush count, and what subjects had been told about the trial. Women were aware not only that they would receive either an active or inert preparation initially, but they also knew that these would be alternated after three months. Obviously when hot flushes did not continue to improve in the second three months for women initially receiving oestrogen, they would realise their treatment sequence, thereby compromising the double blind condition.

Overall, of the eleven symptoms included in the index, only hot flushes showed a significant proportional, but not absolute reduction in response to oestrogen compared with placebo. The authors conclude that 'the definite placebo response of all symptoms in this double blind trial makes it difficult to assess the genuine pharmacological value of short term oestrogen treatment' (p.142).

Fedor-Freybergh (1977)

A controlled study, in which a beneficial effect of oestrogen on all psychological symptoms in comparison with placebo was reported, is that by Fedor-Freybergh (1977). In this trial a small group of women, 11 in all, was compared with a placebo group of 10 women, using a double blind administration. To assess symptomatic outcome, a variety of measures were used, including the Hamilton Depression Scale and two other scales, one to assess general symptoms the other psychological distress. The authors found an improvement in all these scales for the oestrogen group only, thereby apparently indicating a clear effect of oestrogen on psychic functions. This indeed is the only trial in which such a widespread effect of oestrogen on psychological symptoms has been found. However a curious omission in this trial is the absence of any reference to vasomotor symptoms. Again it could well be that the overall improvement in psychological wellbeing in those receiving oestrogen, is secondary to the relief of hot flushes.

Campbell and Whitehead (1977)

A study which throws light on this issue is that by Campbell and Whitehead (1977), which is also the best designed and most comprehensive controlled trial to date. This study consisted of two double blind crossover trials of conjugated equine oestrogen against placebo. One trial ran for four months the other for twelve months. In all 24 symptoms were assessed using visual analogue scales, women selected for the short trial having much more severe symptoms initially. In the four month trial, oestrogen produced a significantly greater improvement than placebo on the central symptoms of hot flushes and two other oestrogen linked symptoms, vaginal dryness and urinary frequency. Of the remaining 21 symptoms, nine, mostly psychological ones, also showed a significantly greater improvement with oestrogen than placebo. These nine symptoms are listed in Table 2.2. There was also a highly significant placebo effect on five symptoms (vaginal dryness, urinary frequency, memory, skin appearance and coital satisfaction).

A repeated objection to interpreting such findings as indicating a direct psychic effect of oestrogen has been that such improvements could

Table 2.2

*Symptoms Improved by Oestrogen
Therapy when Compared with Placebo*

4 Month Study	12 Month Study
Hot flushes	Hot flushes
Vaginal dryness *	Vaginal dryness
Urinary frequency	Urinary frequency
Poor memory *	Poor memory
Anxiety *	Insomnia
Worry about age *	
Worry about self *	
Irritability	
Insomnia	
Headaches	
Optimism	
Good spirits	

* Improved in patients without hot flushes
Adapted from Campbell and Whitehead (1977)

be due to what is sometimes referred to as a 'domino' effect, arising from the invariable relief from vasomotor symptoms and/or atrophic vaginitis. In this particular study however, 20 women were experiencing no vasomotor symptoms. When these women's responses were examined it was found that improvement with oestrogen therapy was observed for only four of the nine psychological symptoms which had originally responded to oestrogen. These were poor memory, anxiety and worry about self and age. This provides good evidence that improvement in the other five symptoms was conditional on improvement of the vasomotor ones. The authors contend that the improvement in memory and anxiety in these 20 women suggests that a 'mental tonic' effect also exists and occurs independent of change in vasomotor symptoms. However, it could be argued that the improvement in these symptoms was also due to a domino effect arising from relief of vaginal dryness (atrophic vaginitis), which also improved in this group (see Table 2.2 again).

Turning to the twelve month trial, the pattern of improvement in symptoms was slightly different for both oestrogen and placebo. Although oestrogen was still more effective in reducing hot flushes, vaginal dryness and urinary frequency, it now benefited only two (insomnia and poor memory) of the nine symptoms improved in the shorter trial, and this to a lesser degree. These are also shown in Table 2.2. The authors suggest that this decreased response to oestrogen was due to women in the twelve month trial having less severe symptoms than those in the four month trial. This may be correct but an additional factor could have been that over the longer period of time the domino effect arising from relief of hot flushes wears off, and some psychological symptoms return.

A further finding of interest in this study was that in the twelve month trial no significant difference emerged between the effects of oestrogen and placebo on two standardised scales for assessing psychiatric symptoms. These were the Beck Depression Inventory and the General Hospital Questionnaire (Goldberg, 1972). The authors conclude that these scales are probably not sufficiently sensitive to monitor changes in the psychological status of postmenopausal women, most of whom do not have a psychiatric disorder. While this may be correct for the first of these scales it is certainly not true of the latter, many of the items of which are to be found among the symptomatology of menopausal women (see study by Ballinger in section 3.2).

Dennerstein, Burrows, Hyman and Sharpe (1979)

Another study which lends some support to the domino effect hypothesis is that by Dennerstein et al. (1979). These authors compared three active preparations with placebo in a double blind crossover trial. The active preparations consisted of an oestrogen (ethinyloestradiol), a progestogen (norgestrel) and a preparation containing both. Each woman received each treatment for three months. Oestrogen by itself proved to be the most effective in reducing scores on the Hamilton Depression Rating Scale, but further analysis revealed that this was mainly due to a decrease in the anxiety items of this scale, that is, the less severe symptoms. Six other symptoms, general feeling of wellbeing, mood, irritability, anxiety, fatigue and insomnia were also individually assessed. Although the placebo and progestogen almost invariably had the least effect on these, only insomnia was significantly reduced by oestrogen, in comparison with placebo, by the end of the three month period. Three other symptoms were also self rated by women using a visual analogue method, but no significant differences emerged between any treatments for these.

The authors then went onto consider the extent to which change in the Hamilton Scale reflected the alleviation of hot flushes, as virtually all women in the study had shown some relief from these (Dennerstein et al., 1978). This was done statistically by means of an analysis of co-variance to determine whether the reducation in the Hamilton Depression Scores could be accounted for by the reduction in hot flushes. A considerable decline in significance levels demonstrated that this was indeed the case. Nevertheless, the finding of a significant residual improvement in mood, once the effect of hot flushes had been excluded, led the authors to conclude that there was some evidence to support a beneficial psychotropic effect of oestrogen. However, the use of a statistical device is not entirely satisfactory, and the procedure of Campbell and Whitehead (1977) in comparing women with and without hot flushes is clearly a more acceptable way of demonstrating a domino effect or otherwise.

A study, although not a controlled one, which is also relevant to the domino effect hypothesis is that of Chakravarti et al. (1979). These authors compared a group of women, attending a menopausal clinic, who were experiencing hot flushes together with other symptoms, with a similar group not experiencing hot flushes. Both groups received conjugated equine oestrogen over a six month period. Relief from other symptoms (depression, headaches, irritability etc.) in those women initially reporting hot flushes was on average three times greater than in those not reporting such symptoms. As the study was not a controlled one, any improvement in symptoms in women not experiencing flushes could have been due to a placebo effect. This study therefore illustrates once again that most of the improvement in non-vasomotor symptoms may be secondary to relief from hot flushes.

Schiff, Regestein, Tulchinsky and Ryan (1979)

A clinical trial, the results of which could be seen as concurring with this explanation in regard to the symptom of insomnia is that by Schiff et al. (1979). As in the study by Thomson and Oswald (1977), sleep was assessed objectively in a laboratory set up in a double blind crossover trial of conjugated oestrogen against placebo. In addition to sleep measures, daily hot flush counts were made and women also rated themselves daily on nine other symptoms over the trial period. Symptoms included sweating, vaginal irritation and dryness, breakthrough bleeding, breast pains, tiredness, dizziness, headaches and nausea. Of the ten symptoms hot flushes alone were significantly lessened by oestrogen therapy.

Oestrogen also had a beneficial effect on sleep, particularly sleep latency, and it increased REM sleep but not length of sleep. Thus, symptomatically the effects of oestrogen were once again on vasomotor symptoms only. The finding in regard to sleep is consistent with that of Thomson and Oswald (1977), on this occasion with a different preparation. It could be that oestrogens in general have a sedative effect, but for this trial the most parsimonious explanation is that the improved quality, but not length of sleep, is a result of relief from the nocturnal disturbance caused by vasomotor symptoms.

Paterson (1982)

Another study in which the effects of oestrogen on non-vasomotor was found to be largely limited to insomnia is that by Paterson (1982). In this double blind crossover trial a preparation containing both oestrogen (ethinyloestradiol) and progestogen (norethisterone) was compared with a placebo over a three month period. Outcome was assessed by, in all, 23 symptoms, each rated in severity, plus a measure of weekly hot flush count. There was a highly significant reduction in both the number and severity of hot flushes and the severity of sweating at all durations of active therapy, the placebo effect being fairly small. As far as the other 21 symptoms were concerned there was a slight improvement in insomnia and to a lesser extent in loss of confidence and lack of energy, but these improvements occurred only in those women receiving the active preparation first. A further indication that the active preparation had little effect on symptoms, apart from the vasomotor ones, was that although there was a highly significant difference in the reduction of total symptoms scores between the drug and placebo, this disappeared when hot flushes and sweats were removed from this measure. Thus the author concluded that 'oestrogen deficiency had only a poor association with many of these symptoms' (p.92).

An interesting feature of this crossover study is that for the group of women who received the active preparation for three months, followed by the placebo for three months, the insomnia measure exactly followed the monthly pattern of the vasomotor symptoms, with gradual improvement followed by gradual worsening. This is consistent with the suggestion made at the end of the previous study that the vasomotor symptoms are aetiologically linked to the quality of sleep.

Nordin, Jones, Crilly, Marshall and Brooke (1980)

Like Dennerstein et al. (1979) these authors also compared ethinyloestradiol with a progestogen (norethisterone) and a placebo, this time in a double blind controlled trial. Using an 18 symptom checklist it was found that total symptom scores fell in both active therapies but that there was no significant change in the placebo group. Unfortunately, no details are presented for individual symptoms but the authors report that most of the improvement in total symptom scores was due to a reduction in hot flushes. The placebo effect in this study was minimal, perhaps, as the authors suggest, because the inclusion of the placebo in this trial was explained to women in advance. These authors conclude, contrary to Dennerstein et al. (1978), that the particular progestogen used in this trial was almost as effective as oestrogen in alleviating menopausal symptoms.

Ikeda and Colleagues (1978)

In the final controlled trial to be described, that by Ikeda et al. (1978), conjugated equine oestrogen was compared with placebo in a straight double blind comparison. Outcome was evaluated, somewhat inadequately, by means of an overall judgement by a clinician and the patient herself, as to whether treatment had been effective or not. No difference emerged between oestrogen and placebo for either the clinician's or patient's judgements, the majority of patients in both groups having improved. An interesting finding however, was that when women were subdivided as to whether they were psychologically normal or abnormal on the basis of personality tests, oestrogen was significantly more effective in those women classified as psychologically normal. The likely explanation of this is that alleviation of hot flushes would be unlikely to have any marked domino effect on women with very severe psychological symptoms.

A similar finding was reported by Schneider et al. (1977) in a study, which although again not a controlled trial, is of some relevance to this review. This study consisted simply of a comparison of 20 menopausal women with respect to their mean scores on the Beck Depression Inventory, before and after a month on conjugated equine oestrogen. The relevance of this study lies in the generally negative outcome as there was no change in depression scores for the group as a whole. There was however, some suggestion that women who were less depressed showed a slight improvement which was not significant. This could either have been a placebo effect, which may not have shown up in severely depressed women or alternatively, as in the study by Ikeda et al. (1978), because of the failure of hot flush relief to have any effect on more disturbed women. This would imply that even the domino effect is restricted to minor symptoms. The overall finding is also consistent with that of Campbell and Whitehead (1977), George et al. (1973) and Coppen and Wood (1978) regarding the ineffectiveness of oestrogen on depression, as measured by the Beck Inventory.

The outcome of each trial in regard to which symptoms or measures were significantly more alleviated by oestrogen than placebo, is summarised in the final column of Table 2.1.

2.4. PSYCHOTROPIC EFFECTS OF OESTROGEN

Much has been written in the literature about the beneficial psychological effects of oestrogen replacement (see section 2.2). In this section we shall address ourselves specifically to this assertion, in the light of the findings of the clinical trials which have just been reviewed and other evidence. The four issues which have repeatedly arisen in the preceding review of clinical trials on which the question of the direct psychotropic effect of oestrogen centres are, the strength of the placebo effect, the effect of oestrogen on individual psychological symptoms, the strength of the domino effect and the existence of a 'mental tonic' effect. A fifth issue is, what effect oestrogen has on psychological functioning as assessed by psychometric and personality tests. These five issues will now be considered in this section, the first half of which consists mainly of a drawing together of what has been said in section 2.3. in relation to each study separately.

Strength of the Placebo Effect

Symptoms of a psychological nature can of course be alleviated by procedures other than direct pharmacological agents, and in particular show a highly variable response to placebo. This was apparent from the outset in the foregoing review of clinical trials. In neither of the first two trials reviewed was oestrogen shown to have much effect on psychological symptoms over and above a placebo response. This was because in one trial (Martin et al., 1971) neither oestrogen nor placebo improved such symptoms, whereas in the second (Jarvinen et al., 1971) the improvement following oestrogen therapy was offset by the large placebo effect. These latter authors accounted for this by the fact that their subjects came from a remote rural area of Finland and were paid the cost of travel and a daily allowance. From the results of two later studies, one by Coope et al. (1975) in which the placebo response was extremely large, the other by Nordin et al. (1980) in which it was minimal, it was apparent that the strength of the placebo effect could also depend on what exactly women were told about the design of the trial, and in particular the type of placebo procedure to be used. Ikeda et al. (1978) and Schneider et al. (1977) also noted that oestrogen had a greater influence on milder than more severe symptoms, a finding which would also be consistent with a placebo response.

Variations in the strength of the placebo effect can therefore be attributed to the varying conditions under which trials are carried out, as well as to differences in subjects. It has been suggested that blind placebo controlled trials of oestrogen are impossible to carry out because of the obvious and rapid effect the active preparation has on vasomotor symptoms. This need not necessarily always be the case however. As at least three of the trials revealed (Jarvinen et al., 1971; Thomson and Oswald, 1977; Strickler et al., 1977), when the placebo response is exceptionally large, the inert placebo can have an effect on vasomotor symptoms equal to that of the active preparation. In certain circumstances therefore, a placebo appears to be capable of improving all types of climacteric symptoms equally.

Individual Psychological Symptoms

Aylward (1973) claimed that oestrogen had a specific effect on depression as measured by the Hamilton Rating Scale, a finding which Thomson and Oswald (1977) failed to substantiate in a similar but better designed and better analysed study. This negative finding received some confirmation from an oestrogen trial by Coppen and Wood (1978) with psychiatrically depressed women. George et al. (1973) were also unable to distinguish the effect of oestrogen from placebo on a wide range of 'minor psychiatric' symptoms. Other researchers who have obtained similar results in regard to individual psychological symptoms were Jarvinen et al. (1971), Utian (1972a), Strickler et al. (1977) and Schiff et al. (1979), while Martin et al. (1971) and Paterson (1982) found any such effect to be limited to one or two symptoms only. Thus in the majority of the above clinical trials, in which the effect of oestrogen on individual psychological symptoms has been examined, no specific psychotropic effect has been found, in excess of a placebo response (see final column Table 2.1). Apart from Aylward's work, however, an exception to this is that of Fedor-Freybergh (1977) who found oestrogen to have a beneficial effect on all the measures of psychological symptoms and functioning employed. No reference was made in this study to vasomotor symptoms, which brings in the issue of the domino effect on psychological symptoms.

The Domino Effect

Campbell and Whitehead (1977) convincingly demonstrated that any improvement in individual psychological symptoms when it did occur was, in the main, a result of a domino effect arising from the alleviation of hot flushes, a finding confirmed by Chakravarti et al. (1979) and Dennerstein et al. (1978). The latter, however, did conclude that there was a residual direct psychotropic effect of oestrogen on depression when the effect of the alleviation of vasomotor symptoms on depression was partialled out statistically. Methodologically, however, this technique is inferior to that used by Campbell and Whitehead.

The 'Mental Tonic' Effect

The idea that oestrogen has a generalised 'mental tonic' effect was introduced by Utian (1972b), who, like others, found oestrogen to have no effect on individual psychological symptoms (Utian, 1972a). This was based on improvement in an overall clinical rating of the woman's feeling of general wellbeing following oestrogen. However, the particular trial in which this was found was a single blind one, and in two later double blind trials, neither Strickler et al. (1977), nor Ikeda et al. (1978) were able to confirm this general effect, using a similar measure of overall wellbeing.

Psychological Test Performance

There have been a number of empirical studies in which the effect of oestrogen on certain mental functions and personality characteristics have been assessed using objective psychometric measures. Rauramo et al. (1975), for example, compared two groups of oophorectomised women, one of which received no treatment the other an oestrogen preparation (oestradiol valerate), with regard to their performance on tests of memory, logical memory, reaction time and speed of performance. No differences on these measures emerged between these groups over a six month period. However, the non-treatment group complained of more subjective symptoms, including poor memory and loss of concentration. The failure of improvement in these subjective complaints to be reflected in objective test performance once again suggests the presence of a placebo or possibly a domino effect on self reported symptoms. It should be noted that this was not a blind trial, as the control group received no treatment.

A similar type of study, and one which is often quoted as providing evidence for a beneficial effect of oestrogen on mental functioning (e.g. in Gerdes et al., 1982) is one by Vanhulle and Demol (1976). The subjects, all nuns living in a religious community, were randomly allocated to an oestrogen and a placebo control group using a double blind administration. The trial period was three months and each woman was tested on a wide variety of objective tasks before and after treatment. These tasks included measures of visual and auditory memory, concentration, learning ability, reaction time, alertness, tempo of work and attention. A significant difference emerged between the two groups at post treatment on only one of these measures, that of attention. Thus, oestrogen in fact did little to improve mental functioning of this group of menopausal nuns in any general way. A not dissimilar outcome was reported by Herrmann et al. (1978), using on this occasion a group of twelve healthy male subjects. The psychological performance tests included critical flicker fusion, reaction time to light and sound, pegboard test, a speed of tapping test and an arithmetical exercise. Apart from the tapping test, the performance of the oestrogen group was no different from that of the placebo group.

A fourth study however, did find changes on a number of different objective measures of psychological functioning in a group of women receiving oestrogen. This was again the study by Fedor-Freybergh (1977), previously referred to, in which, over a three month period, women receiving oestrogen showed significant improvement on tests of choice reaction time, visual search, concentration and attention compared with a placebo group which showed no change. However, as has already been pointed out (section 2.3) no reference is made in this study to the severity of hot flushes nor the extent to which these were alleviated by oestrogen. It is not inconceivable that, as with subjective symptoms, performance on such tests could be substantially improved if women were no longer experiencing these distressing symptoms.

Changes on personality tests have also been examined in a number of the clinical trials of oestrogen referred to in the previous section, almost invariably with negative results. As noted earlier Strickler et al. (1977) found no evidence of changes in personality, using the Minnesota Multiphasic Personality Inventory, following oestrogen, a finding which confirmed that of an earlier uncontrolled study by Bolding and Willicut

(1969), using the same test. Campbell and Whitehead (1977) in their double blind crossover trial found an equally significant improvement in the Neuroticism Dimension of the Eysenck Personality Inventory after both oestrogen and placebo but no changes in Extraversion. In contrast, Fedor-Freybergh (1977) again found oestrogen changed both these personality characteristics but the placebo did not. This last study is unique among clinical trials in that oestrogen appeared to improve all aspects of psychological functioning — symptoms, cognitive processes and personality traits and, as shall be seen in section 4.2, sexual functioning — whereas placebo had no such effect. Finally Schiff et al. (1979) included in their assessment three personality scales, the Clyde Mood Adjective Checklist, the Gottschalk-Gleser Test and the Minnesota Multiphasic Personality Inventory. These tests assess in all some 26 attributes of personality but in only two of these were any changes observed. Following oestrogen women became less outwardly aggressive but more inwardly hostile. How this is to be interpreted the authors do not say.

It has been previously mentioned that one of the claims made for oestrogen therapy is that it slows down the ageing process. Only one empirical study exists in this area, and is often quoted (e.g. in Kopera, 1973; Fedor-Freybergh, 1977; Lauritzen and van Keep, 1978) as objective evidence that oestrogen can indeed act to retard the decline in personality with age. This is the study reported in Kantor et al. (1968) and Michael et al. (1970). These authors followed up a group of women between the ages 59 and 91 years, living in a residential home for the elderly over a three year period. Half the women received oestrogen and the other half placebo, in a double blind administration. Patients were rated at regular intervals by nurses using the Hospital Adjustment Scale, an instrument designed to measure a number of facets of behaviour within a hospital setting.

The authors concluded that over the three year period, women on oestrogen maintained a higher level of personality functioning than did those receiving placebo. A close examination of the data of this study however, makes this conclusion somewhat difficult to accept. At the outset, for reasons not explained, women receiving oestrogen had higher levels of adaptation than did those who were to receive the placebo. Thus, women on placebo were functioning at a poor level from the start of the trial, and this could have prevented any placebo response taking place. Also the drop out rate over the three year period was excessively high. Only one third remained in each group at the end of the three year period. Furthermore, the drop out rate was 60 per cent in the oestrogen group at the end of the first year, compared with 25 per cent in the placebo group over the same period. These initial differences between subjects in the placebo and oestrogen groups, and the large and differential drop out rates, make this study a difficult one to evaluate.

In a later study, Kantor et al. (1978) followed up a similar group of women over a one year period in which the group of institutionalised women were compared with a group living in the community. Both groups received conjugated oestrogen, but as no placebo control group was included the trial was not a blind one. As in the previous study the drop out was high at 46 per cent. Only the institutionalised subjects showed any clear improvement over the trial period on a number of symptoms and personality measures. The authors offer no explanation for this differential response and again this is a difficult study to evaluate. It could be that elderly women in institutions are more prone to placebo effects. On balance therefore, evidence for a beneficial effect of oestrogen on the cognitive functioning or personality of women, as assessed by objective psychological tests, is negative or at best equivocal.

Finally, in this section, it is necessary to refer briefly to three other uncontrolled oestrogen therapy trials, in all three of which claims are made for a direct psychotropic effect of oestrogen. First, Durst and Maoz (1979), on the basis of the greater improvement in psychological wellbeing of a group of 40 women who completed a year's treatment of conjugated oestrogen, in comparison with a group of 40 women who began but dropped out of therapy within three months, concluded that the psychotropic effects of oestrogen had been confirmed! A similar claim for 'the psychotherapeutic effect of oestrogen substitution' was made in a paper of that title by Wenderlein (1980). In this paper Wenderlein reports a beneficial effect of oestrogen on a number of personality and symptom measures. As there was no control group, placebo effect cannot be determined nor consequently were either patient or doctor blind. Furthermore, in all, 455 women were initially considered for the trial and of these 161 (35 per cent) started on therapy and 64 (14 per cent) completed the trial. Clearly no sound conclusions can be derived from an uncontrolled study of such a highly selected population.

In the third study Gerdes et al. (1982) concluded that their results provide 'statistical confirmation that oestrogen replacement therapy is associated with attenuation of psychological symptoms, notably depression and anxiety' (p.102). This conclusion was based on the finding that, of 18 psychological measures, oestrogen produced a significantly greater improvement on half these measures than did clonidine. Two criticisms can be made of this study. No placebo group was included, hence the reason for it not featuring among controlled trials listed in Table 2.1. The trial, in effect, consisted of a straight comparison between conjugated equine oestrogen and clonidine over a 20 week period in two groups of postmenopausal women. The so-called control group consisted of a group of *a*symptomatic women who received *no* treatment whatsoever. Furthermore, and more importantly, no reference is made to vasomotor symptoms in this report, so that any possible domino effect cannot be ascertained. This, despite the fact that in a previous paper on the same study the authors reported that oestrogen was effective in reducing hot flushes whereas clonidine was not (Sonnendecker and Polakow, 1980). The definitive conclusions of the authors of these three studies as to the psychological effects of oestrogen replacement, can scarcely be justified on the basis of these inadequate designs.

This raises an important point regarding the consideration which should be given to each of the studies so far reviewed, in weighing up the evidence for and against a direct psychotropic effect of oestrogen. In doing this, that of Campbell and Whitehead (1977) must clearly be seen as of critical importance. This is the only properly controlled study in which it has been possible to directly assess the magnitude of the effect the relief of vasomotor symptoms has on other symptoms. This study has shown this effect to be a powerful one, as, of a total of 21 symptoms, in only two was there any significant improvement in the *absence* of a decline in vasomotor symptoms, and indeed it could be argued that the improvement in those two symptoms was secondary to a reduction in the symptoms of atrophic vaginitis. A direct psychotropic effect of oestrogen on climacteric women's psychological symptoms, cognitive functioning or personality in general, remains to be demonstrated.

2.5. SUMMARY AND CONCLUSION

In the first section of this chapter we saw how diverse clinical opinion was regarding those climacteric symptoms which could be accounted for by oestrogen deficiency. We have seen similar diverse views expressed over the years regarding the efficacy of oestrogen replacement and in particular its effect on psychological symptoms and wellbeing. At least some of this diversity of views can be attributed to the wide variation and, in many instances, inadequacies in the methodology of clinical trials of oestrogen therapy in early years. Even the controlled trials carried out over the past decade vary in a variety of ways in regard to the design of the trial, the types of oestrogen preparations used, the size of the sample, the type of patients, the time period over which effects are evaluated, and finally with regard to how outcome is assessed and the data analysed (see Table 2.1). Such diversity in method must inevitably lead to some differences in outcome and interpretation of results. Nevertheless, despite these variations in method it is possible, on the basis of a close examination of the existing research, to make a number of general points regarding their outcome.

1. All trials show that oestrogen therapy reduces vasomotor symptoms and, where they have been assessed, the symptoms of atrophic vaginitis. However, in at least three trials (Thomson and Oswald, 1977; Jarvinen et al., 1971; Strickler et al., 1977) this improvement in vasomotor symptoms was not substantially greater than that for the placebo. Trials vary considerably in regard to the strength of the placebo effect on vasomotor symptoms, in some it is non-existent, in others modest and in other quite large and equal to that of the active preparation.

2. Many trials have shown an improvement in some other somatic and psychological symptoms as a result of oestrogen therapy, but this improvement is invariably much less than that of vasomotor symptoms. Furthermore, in almost all trials, the improvement in most of these other symptoms in response to oestrogen is not much greater than that for placebo. The strength of the placebo effect in any particular trial appears to be a function of the specific conditions of the trial. Where the double blind condition is effectively maintained, the placebo effect is large.

3. In trials in which the effect of oestrogen on non-vasomotor symptoms has been significantly greater than for placebo, this has occurred with one exception for one or two symptoms only, and there is no consistency, except perhaps for insomnia, as to which symptoms are so affected across trials (see final column Table 2.1). In the case of improved sleep, the most likely explanation is that this is due to the alleviation of nocturnal sweating.

4. The one exception to the above is the study by Campbell and Whitehead (1977) in which a number of symptoms, in all nine, responded significantly better to oestrogen than to placebo. For most of these symptoms, however, this was demonstrably a result of relief from vasomotor symptoms. This domino effect has been confirmed by two other researchers — Dennerstein et al. (1979) and Chakravarti et al. (1979).

5. Claims that oestrogen has a beneficial psychotropic effect has on the whole been unsubstantiated, there being little convincing or consistent evidence that it either improves individual psychological symptoms or has a general mental tonic effect in addition to the above mentioned placebo or domino effects.
6. The effect of oestrogen on psychological functioning in general, as measured by performance and personality tests, is conflicting with the balance of evidence indicating little or no effect.

Conclusion

Despite the variation in methodology and details of outcome, there does seem to be a general consensus regarding the main focus of interest of this chapter, namely, the effect of oestrogen replacement on climacteric symptoms, other than vasomotor ones and those of atrophic vaginitis. The answer would seem to be that there is very little consistent evidence that these other non-specific symptoms can be directly improved by oestrogen treatment. Any such observed effect is most parsimoniously ascribed to a placebo or domino effect, arising from relief of hot flushes and atrophic vaginitis. Nor, for the same reasons, does oestrogen therapy appear to have any direct effect on women's general psychological wellbeing or functioning.

Nevertheless, the notion that oestrogen has a beneficial effect on the psychological functioning of climacteric women is still perpetuated over the years in reviews such as those of Kopera (1973), Fedor-Freybergh (1977), Lauritzen and van Keep (1978) and Greenblatt et al. (1980); in clinical reports by Moore et al. (1975) and Studd et al. (1977a); and in uncontrolled trials such as those by Durst and Maoz (1979), Wenderlein (1980) and Gerdes et al. (1982). It must therefore be emphatically stated that, on the basis of the available evidence, oestrogen does not appear to have any *direct* nor substantial effect on symptoms or functions of climacteric women, other than those which there is good reason to suppose are a consequence of oestrogen deficiency. In particular, any psychotropic effect of oestrogen remains undemonstrated. The answer to the question posed in the introduction to this chapter is that only symptoms of vasomotor instability and atrophic vaginitis can be confidently attributed to oestrogen deficiency.

3

Symptoms During the Climacteric among Women in the General Population

In Chapter 2 we were concerned with establishing which of the many symptoms women experience during the climacteric could be directly accounted for by hormonal changes. It was concluded that only vasomotor symptoms and those of atrophic vaginitis could be attributed directly to decreased oestrogen production. In this chapter we proceed to examine the role of one of the other potential sources of climacteric symptoms, depicted in Figure 1.2, namely the event of the menopause. To do this however, we must obtain some idea of the degree and nature of climacteric symptomatology among women in general, as opposed to those attending gynaecological or menopausal clinics, or participating in drugs trials. Inevitably these groups are self selective and therefore probably unrepresentative of the population of climacteric women as a whole. Several reports from different countries in the world have indicated that levels of psychopathology among women attending gynaecological clinics can be extremely high. In studies by Munro (1969) in Scotland, Sainsbury (1960) in England, Worsley et al. (1977) in Australia, Indira and Murthy (1980a) in India and Ballinger (1977) again in Scotland, estimates of 'psychiatric morbidity' among such women have ranged from 10 per cent in the case of the first, to as much as 53 per cent in the case of the last named study. While data gathered from such groups may be valid for certain purposes, for example, to evaluate the efficacy of oestrogen replacement, for others they are clearly not.

Therefore, as has been said above, in order to gain some idea of the degree and nature of climacteric symptoms, and their temporal association to the menopause, we must turn to those surveys of climacteric symptomatology which have been carried out using general or 'normal' population samples of women. A review of these surveys forms the substance of this chapter.

3.1. SURVEYS OF SYMPTOMS

Surveys of symptoms among the general population of climacteric women have been carried out only within the past two decades. The one exception is a very early survey conducted in the late 1920s by the Medical Women's Federation of Great Britain, later published in *The Lancet* (Council of the Medical Women's Federation, 1933). This survey is largely of historical interest, as it is difficult to compare it with more modern surveys because of its methodological differences and inadequacies. The sample of 1000 women was scarcely representative of women in general, as according to the authors many of them were living in public assistance institutions in different parts of the British Isles. The criterion for selection was that five years or more had elapsed since the cessation of menses, yet, somewhat surprisingly, their ages ranged from 29 to 91 years. Many of these women must therefore have been recalling their menopausal experiences over a lengthy period of time. Nevertheless, of some interest is the finding that only some 10 per cent of this nonclinical population reported themselves as having been 'incapacitated' by the menopause. The authors conclude that 'in view of the general impression acquired from the literature on the subject it was somewhat surprising that approximately 900 of 1000 unselected women stated that they had carried out their daily routine tasks without a single interruption due to menopausal symptoms' (p.106).

Further general population surveys did not in fact begin to appear until the mid 1960s, when in 1965, Neugarten and Kraines published their influential survey of 'menopausal symptoms' in women of various ages in the United States. This was followed over the next 15 years by in all 13 similar surveys from other countries. Details of all 14 surveys can be found in Table 3.1, which summarises the methodology of each. The common feature of most of these surveys is that they are attempts to determine the prevalence of various symptoms in general population samples of climacteric women, who are currently experiencing or who have just experienced the menopause, sometimes referred to as the perimenopause, in comparison with those who are either pre or postmenopausal. In this way it is hoped to establish what symptons, if any, are typical of, or at least common at the time of the menopause. In general, it has been found that all symptoms commonly assessed are reported not only among women of similar ages who are not menopausal, but are commonly reported by women of other ages. The task is therefore one of determining whether or not there are certain symptoms which are experienced moreso by women during the perimenopause than at other times.

As can be seen in Table 3.1 researchers diverge widely in regard to the various methods employed in performing this task. For example, there are wide differences between surveys in regard to the degree of randomness and size of the sample and the age range investigated. The majority of studies are confined to the climacteric period, taken usually to be the fourth and fifth decades, although there is some variation as to the exact age limits of this period. In all cases the response rate is in excess of 70 per cent, which is consistent with that usually obtained in other types of general population surveys. The data has been gathered either by means of a postal questionnaire, sent out to the subject, or by personal interview, usually conducted at the subject's home. The latter, if conducted properly, is generally a more superior method.

Variation, however, in three aspects of methodology, namely, operational definitions of menopausal status, the methods of assessing symptoms and the form of reporting results, make any detailed comparison of the outcome of more than two surveys at a time difficult. Although for the most part, the method of the last menstrual cycle has

Table 3.1
Summary of the Method of General Population Surveys of Symptoms During the Climacteric

Authors	Location	Source of Sample	Size and Age	Response Rate	Method of Data Collection	Menopausal Status	Method of Assessing Symptoms
Neugarten and Kraines (1965)	Chigaco, USA	Mothers of school pupils	460 13—64	—	Personal interview	Self defined	28 symptom checklist
Jaszmann et al. (1969b)	Ede, Holland	All middle aged women	2923 40—60	71%	Postal questionnaire	Jaszmann's criteria	13 symptom checklist
Rybo and Westerberg (1971)	Goteborg, Sweden	Community registar	1462 38—60	90%	—	Menstrual cycle	8 symptom checklist
Thomson et al. (1973)	Aberdeen, Scotland	GP lists	269 40—60	92%	Postal questionnaire	McKinlay's criteria	12 symptom checklist
McKinlay and Jefferys (1974)	London, England	GP lists	538 45—54	95%	Postal questionnaire	McKinlay's criteria	8 symptom checklist
Sharma and Saxena (1981)	Varanasi, India	Clubs, schools, personal contact	405 40—55	—	Personal interview	Jaszmann's criteria	33 symptom checklist
Ballinger (1975)	Dundee, Scotland	GP lists	539 40—55	71%	Postal questionnaire	McKinlay's criteria	General hospital questionnaire
Van Keep and Kellerhals (1974, 1975)	Zurich, Switzerland	Random-route sampling	448 41—60	92%	Personal interview	Jaszmann's criteria	Climacteric index
Severne (1979)	Belgium	Random-route sampling	992 46—55	95%	Personal interview	Jaszmann's criteria	Circulatory index, Nervosity index
Greene and Cooke (1980)	Glasgow, Scotland	Electoral roll	230 35—54	85%	Personal interview	McKinlay's criteria	Vasomotor, somatic and psychological scales (factor analysis)
Kaufert and Syrotuik (1981)	Winnipeg, Canada	GP lists	148 not given	74%	Postal questionnaire	Jaszmann's criteria	Vasomotor, and psychological scales (factor analysis)
Mikkelsen and Holte (1982)	Drammen, Norway	Community register	139 45—55	75%	Postal questionnaire	Menstrual cycle	Vasomotor, somatic and psychological scales (factor analysis)
Wood (1979)	Melbourne, Australia	Community survey	948 20—65	85%	Personal interview	Age of menopause	20 symptom checklist
Bungay et al. (1980)	Oxford, England	GP lists	806 30—64	72%	Postal questionnaire	Age of menopause	40 symptom checklist

been used to determine menopausal status (that is whether a woman is pre, peri or postmenopausal) the specific criteria used for classifying women into these categories have varied. In assessing symptoms, most authors have used ad hoc checklists of symptoms, in which the number of items vary considerably, although there is clearly some agreement on what the core symptoms should be. In many instances these symptoms are simply rated, somewhat crudely, as present or absent, with no attempt being made to assess the severity of the symptom. Most authors present their results in the form of percentages of women reporting individual symptoms within each menopausal status group or age group. Others, report the total number of symptoms, or in a few cases the number of different *types* of symptoms experienced, for example, vasomotor, somatic, psychological. These methodological points, together with others, are discussed more fully in Chapter 7. For the present each survey will be reviewed in turn and the salient findings of each noted.

3.2. REVIEW OF SURVEYS

The fourteen surveys summarised in Table 3.1 will be reviewed in the order in which they are listed there, with the object of determining which of the many symptoms, thought to be associated with the climacteric, increase in prevalence at the time of the menopause. In examining this evidence particular attention will be paid in this review to the prevalence of psychological symptoms. As can be seen from Table 3.1, in the first six surveys, results are reported in the form of the prevalence of individual symptoms among women of different menopausal status. In the following six they are reported for the same groups in the form of average scores on specially constructed *scales*, some measuring different types of symptoms. In three of these surveys these scales have been derived from factor analyses of climacteric symptoms. In the final two surveys prevalence of individual symptoms are again reported, but this time within different age bands of adult females. These considerations have determined the order in which surveys are discussed.

Neugarten and Kraines (1965)

The first of these surveys chronologically is that by Neugarten and Kraines (1965). As the title indicates, this consisted of a survey of the reported prevalence of 'menopausal' symptoms over the age range 13 to 64 years. In examining symptoms within such a wide age range, this survey differs from those which were to follow, most of which confine themselves to what would be considered the age range of the climacteric. It is possible therefore in this survey to compare the prevalence of symptoms of menopausal women, not only with adult women who are not menopausal within the climacteric age range (in this case taken as 45 to 54 years), but also with their prevalence in a younger adult women (age range 20 to 44).

The women, all white, were contacted through high schools, women's clubs and church groups within the Chicago Metropolitan area. The sample was therefore in no sense a random one, and according to the authors these women had a higher educational level than the general population. The climacteric women were further divided into whether they were menopausal or non-menopausal on basis of a self evaluation. To assess symptoms a checklist was devised based upon 'careful survey of the medical literature and upon extensive preliminary interviewing. The final form listed the 28 symptoms most often reported by clinicians and by women themselves as being typical or frequent complaints of menopause' (p.267). These symptoms were categorised as to whether they were somatic (e.g. hot flushes, breast pains, aches in the back of the neck and skull), psychosomatic (e.g. headaches, dizzy spells, tired feelings) or psychological (e.g. irritability, crying spells, depression). Each symptom was self rated as present or absent. The full checklist can be found in Table 1.2. The results of this survey are best summarised by considering each of these categories of symptoms.

The average number of each of these types of symptoms for four subgroups within the age range 20 to 54 years are shown in Table 3.2. It should be noted that unlike most surveys to come, pre and postmenopausal women have been grouped together. Although menopausal women had the highest number of all three types of symptoms, significant differences occurred between this group and others only for somatic and psychosomatic symptoms. There were no significant differences between any of the four groups on psychological symptoms. Inspection of the frequency of individual symptoms reveals that the difference between the two climacteric groups was due to the relatively high occurrence of hot flushes and sweating, and to a lesser degree of a few physical symptoms — weight gain, heavy periods and breast pains. The significant difference in psychosomatic symptoms between these two groups was mainly due to one symptom — headaches. Commenting on these results the authors write that 'it is apparent that the somatic and psychosomatic symptoms are reported most often by the menopausal

Table 3.2

Average Number of Symptoms in Relation to Age and Menopausal Status

	20—29 Years	30—44 Years	45—54 Years Pre/Post Menopause	45—54 Years Peri-Menopause
Somatic (includes vasomotor)	3.2	4.1	3.3	5.4
Psychosomatic	2.2	2.3	2.0	2.7
Psychological	4.8	4.5	4.1	5.2

Adapted from Neugarten and Kraines (1965)

women. At the same time, there are only a few scattered instances in which psychologic symptoms were reported significantly more often by the menopausal group than by others' (p.270).

Methodologically, the main weakness of this study is the manner of determining menopausal status. This was done by self evaluation, that is, each woman in the 45 to 54 year age range was asked whether or not she considered herself to be currently passing through the menopause. This is a subjective and unsatisfactory method and clearly may lead to a confounding of symptoms and menopausal status when the women is required to assess both. Later studies have used the more objective method of determining menopausal status according to the time since the last menstrual cycle.

A further criticism is that none of the groups of women was randomly selected. The women in the 45 to 54 years range were mothers of high school graduates and those in other age ranges were contacted through women's clubs and church associations. As such, they cannot be considered as representative of the population at large. This could account for some of the extraordinary high frequency of occurrence of symptoms among these women. To take one example, some 82 per cent of women in the 30 to 44 years age range reported currently feeling irritable and nervous as against 92 per cent in the menopausal group. These remarkably high figures contrast with those reported in future surveys.

For these reasons this is a difficult study to evaluate. However, despite this, perhaps the most striking aspect of this first contemporary survey is its negative findings. That is, what is striking, is the *failure* to find any substantial differences between women who consider themselves to be menopausal, and women of other age groups with regard to psychological symptoms. Indeed, given that women evaluated both menopausal status and symptoms, it might have been anticipated, in view of the common stereotype of the menopause, that symptoms in a group of women reporting themselves as menopausal might have been spuriously high. The relatively low increase in the prevalence of psychological symptoms at the menopause is therefore all the more convincing.

Jaszmann, Van Lith and Zatt (1969b)

In terms of sample size this survey of Dutch women by Jaszmann et al. (1969b) is the largest ever to have been carried out in this field. As the object of the study was the analysis of complaints occurring in women in the general population immediately before, during and after the menopause, the study was restricted to climacteric women, although the age range considered was wider than that used by Neugarten and Kraines for defining the climacteric period. The survey was carried out by means of a postal questionnaire, sent to all women between 40 and 60 years living within the borough of Ede in the Netherlands. The return rate was 71 per cent and data are reported for a total of 2923 women in all. The sample can therefore be considered to be a reasonably random one and representative of the general population.

The authors define the menopause in terms of what they call 'biological age', which in operational terms means defining menopausal status according to menstrual status. This was done as follows:

> Premenopausal — women who reported normal menses during the year preceding the survey.
>
> Menopausal — women reporting a menstrual pattern different from former i.e. those who had more or fewer menstrual flows than previously over the year preceding the survey.
>
> Postmenopausal — women who did not menstruate in the year preceding the survey. This group was further divided into five subgroups according to how long it was since their last period.

This method is clearly superior to the self definition used by Neugarten and Kraines (1965) and is the method used in most subsequent surveys. Symptoms were assessed by means of a 13 item checklist, each symptom being self rated as present or absent.

It was found firstly that the total number of symptoms increased in the menopausal group, and continued to increase for one or two years after the menopause, thereafter declining. However, an analysis of individual symptoms showed that this pattern of temporal relationships to menopausal status did not hold for all symptoms. Indeed, only four symptoms, all physical ones, followed this pattern. These were hot flushes, perspiration, tingling of the extremities, and aches in joints, muscles and bones. These symptoms showed a clear increase at the menopause and continued to rise into the immediate postmenopause. Of these four symptoms, by far the greatest increase in prevalence was in hot flushes. A second group of symptoms, mainly psychological ones, fatigue, headaches, irritability, depression and mental imbalance, slightly increased in prevalence during the menopause, thereafter declining in the immediate postmenopause, having peaked prior to the vasomotor ones. These symptoms, however, were already relatively high in the premenopausal groups and the highest increase of any one of these symptoms was ten per cent. A third group of symptoms, shortness of breath, palpitations, insomnia and dizziness, showed no association with menopausal status whatsoever. An example of each type of pattern of symptoms is illustrated in Figure 3.1, which also shows figures for two

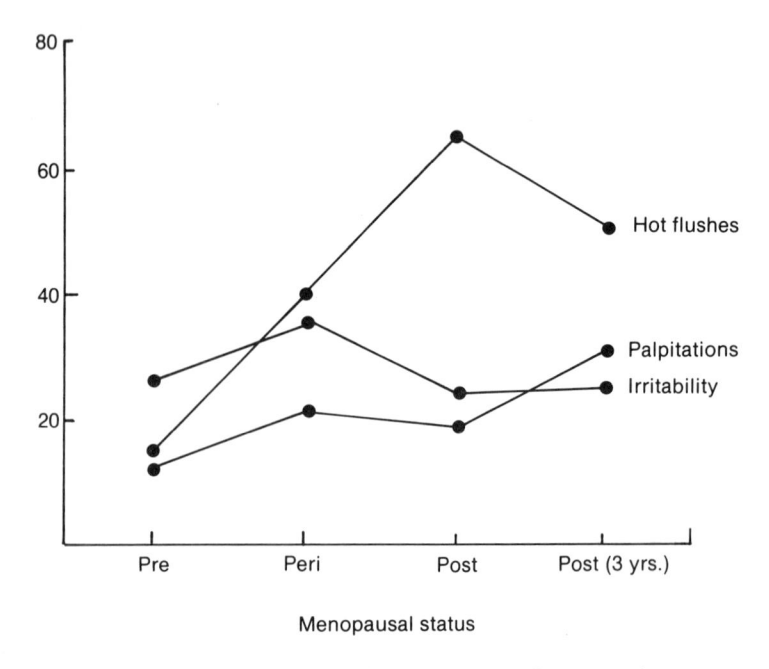

Figure 3.1 Examples of three types of symptom patterns: Percent prevalence. (adapted from Jaszmann et al., 1969b)

years and three years into the postmenopause. Thus of the eleven non-vasomotor symptoms only two followed the same temporal pattern as the vasomotor symptoms. This led the authors to conclude that 'the relationship between frequency of complaints and biological age was compatible with expectations for such complaints in the case of perspiration, tingling sensations of the extremities, and aches in bones, joints and muscles. The compatibility was not found, or found to be a lesser degree, for other complaints' (p.273).

In so far as comparison can be made between the two studies, these findings are not dissimilar to those of Neugarten and Kraines. Both studies show that the increase in symptoms at the menopause is largely confined to an increase in vasomotor symptoms and a few other physical complaints. In both surveys, psychological symptoms are relatively high at the premenopausal stage and show only a marginal increase at the menopause. It should be noted, however, that overall the incidence of various symptoms in all groups is considerably lower in this survey than in that by Neugarten and Kraines. To take only one example, the percentage of menopausal women reporting themselves as feeling depressed in the latter study was 79 per cent against only 25 per cent in this one. These differences may be due to the non-random nature of the sample in the Neugarten and Kraines survey and the more representative nature of Jaszmann's sample.

This Dutch survey is an important one if for no other reason than for the sheer size of the sample of women investigated. It cannot be criticised as being unrepresentative of climacteric women (certainly not Dutch climacteric women) and for that reason its findings with regard to the close temporal association of only two other *physical* symptoms, besides the vasomotor ones, to the menopause must be given serious consideration. The tendency for psychological symptoms to be more frequent in the premenopause than vasomotor symptoms and to peak some time before them, but to a much lesser degree, is also of some significance.

Rybo and Westerberg (1971)

Another fairly large scale investigation of the prevalence of symptoms around the time of the menopause, this time carried out in Sweden, was reported, but not in much detail, by Rybo and Westerberg (1971). The sample consisted of 1462 women in the age range 38 to 60 years, living in the city of Goteberg. The response rate was 90 per cent. Results were reported for a group of postmenopausal women in comparison with a group of younger women having a normal menstrual cycle. Using an eight symptom checklist the two groups were distinguished significantly from each other only in regard to the frequency of hot flushes, there being no differences between the groups in the occurrence of any of the following symptoms; palpitations, pain in back and joints, vertigo, headache, irritability, incontinence and weight gain. These authors concluded 'that with the exception of the hot flushes there was no reason to believe in a specific postmenopausal syndrome' (p.25).

Thompson, Hart and Durno (1973); McKinlay and Jefferys (1974)

The next two surveys, those by Thompson et al. (1973) and McKinlay and Jefferys (1974), were both carried out in the United Kingdom and will be considered together, as the methodology employed in both studies was virtually identical and the conclusions very similar. The object of these studies was not only to determine the prevalence of various symptoms around the time of the menopause, but also to examine the *interrelationships* among the symptoms. The relationships between symptoms and certain sociodemographic factors were also investigated, but discussion of these will be left until a later chapter.

Data for the first study were collected by means of a postal questionnaire sent out to all women aged between 40 and 60 years, who were on the list of a general practice in the outskirts of the city of Aberdeen, Scotland. The total number was 269. In the second survey the population consisted of 538 women aged between 45 and 54 years, whose names were drawn from the registers kept by eight general practices located in or near London. Again a postal questionnaire was used. As can be seen both these studies restrict themselves to the population of climacteric women 'at risk' to the menopause, although the age ranges in each survey differ. In both cases the questionnaire included a short checklist of symptoms, each symptom being self rated on a present/absent basis. A number of questions relating to menstrual history and demographic details were also included. Menopausal status was determined according to last menstrual period using the following criteria previously set out by McKinlay et al. (1972):

> Premenopausal — menstruated within the last three months.
>
> Menopausal — last menstruated between three and twelve months ago.
>
> Postmenopausal — not menustrated within the last twelve months.

In the case of the McKinlay and Jefferys study a transitional group was created, defined as women who had menstruated within the last three months, but with some change in regularity and/or volume in the previous year. This method of classification is, in principle, similar to that of Jaszmann et al. (1969b) but differs in that the perimenopause is defined in terms of when the last period occurred, rather than in terms of irregularity of the menstrual cycle during the preceding year. This would be likely to produce some variation in the classification of women within the premenopausal and menopausal groups (see section 7.2 for a fuller discussion of this point).

In the first of these surveys, that by Thompson et al. (1973), premenopausal and menopausal women were asked if they were currently suffering from any of twelve symptoms, but postmenopausal women were asked if they had suffered from them around the time of the menopause, and not about their current experience. In the event menopausal women were excluded from the reporting of the findings because of their small numbers. It was therefore only possible to compare the prevalence of symptoms reported by premenopausal women with those reported by postmenopausal women retrospectively, that is, when they had been menopausal. This must be considered a somewhat unsatisfactory way of determining symptom prevalence at the menopause. Using such a comparison, the only symptoms on which these two groups were clearly differentiated were the vasomotor ones. No substantial increase was reported at the menopause with regard to depression, headaches, dizzy spells, tiredness, joint pains, bloatedness, backache and swollen ankles. There was however, a tendency for postmenopausal women to report that the symptoms of insomnia and palpitations had increased around the time of the final menses.

In the other study to be considered here, that of McKinlay and Jefferys (1974), it was possible to compare directly the percentages of symptoms currently reported by women within each of the three categories pre, peri and postmenopausal. Eight symptoms were asked about in this survey. With respect to frequency of symptoms only hot flushes and night sweats reached any clear peak in the menopausal group. There was some evidence of lesser increases in the prevalence of insomnia, depression and weight gain, and slight increases in palpitations and dizzy spells, but not headaches, from those regularly menstruating to those who were menopausal. For none of these six symptoms however, was there any clear peak or marked variation at the time of the menopause. In this respect the findings are similar to those of the other United Kingdom study. These effects are summarised in Figure 3.2, which shows a clear peaking of vasomotor symptoms at the menopause, while other symptoms peak some time before this, and to a much lesser degree.

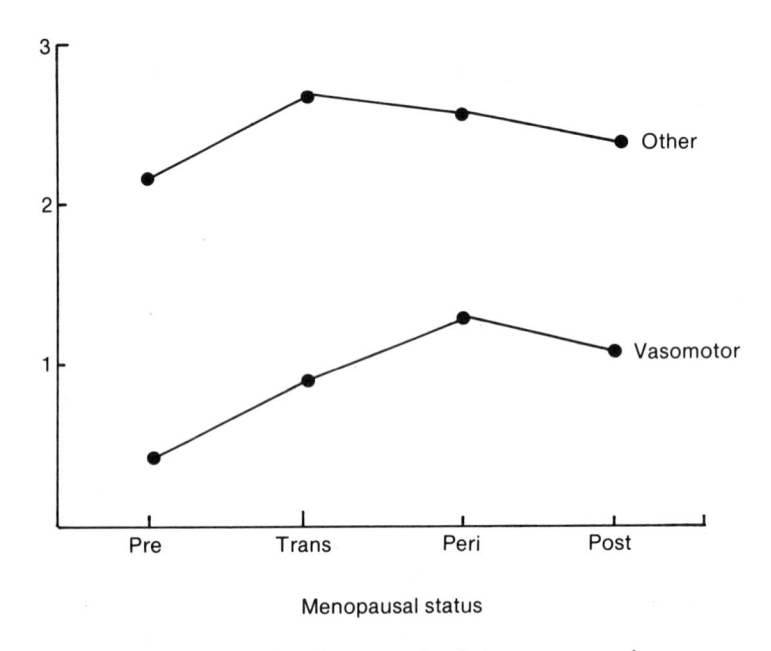

Figure 3.2 Mean number of symptoms in relation to menopausal status. (adapted from McKinlay and Jefferys, 1974)

As indicated above the inter-relationship among symptoms was also examined in both of these surveys. This was done by means of a method of cluster analysis, a statistical technique which allows one to determine which variables form groups or cluster together in two-dimensional space. In both surveys it was confirmed that only hot flushes and night sweats showed any association with menopausal status. The remaining symptoms appeared to be more associated with each other, and formed a loose cluster, relatively distant from vasomotor symptoms and menopausal status. This is illustrated in graphical form in Figure 3.3. Furthermore, when those women within the perimenopausal group, who were experiencing hot flushes, were compared with those who were not, apart from weight increase, there were litle differences between the groups in the occurrence of other symptoms. The conclusion from both these surveys of British women was that 'as far as symptoms are concerned, only the vasomotor disorders, flushing and night sweats, were definitely correlated with menopause' (Thompson et al., 1973, p.71) and that 'the remaining symptoms considered in this survey do not appear to be related to the menopause directly' (McKinlay and Jefferys, 1974, p.114).

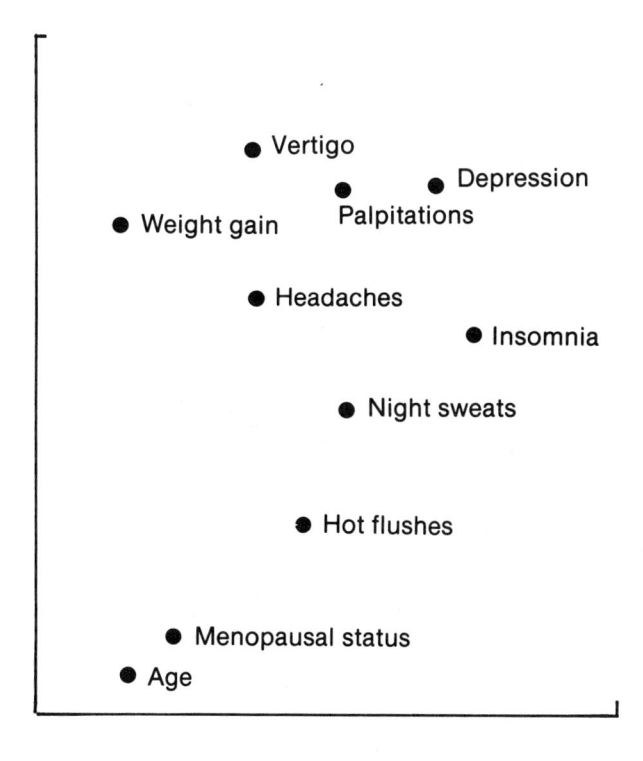

```
                • Vertigo
                        • • Depression
    • Weight gain   Palpitations

            • Headaches
                         • Insomnia

              • Night sweats


            • Hot flushes


       • Menopausal status
      • Age
```

Figure 3.3 Cluster analysis of the relationship between menopausal status and symptoms. (adapted from McKinlay and Jefferys, 1974)

The importance of these two surveys lies in the fact that, using identical methodology, they arrive at similar conclusions regarding the prevalence of different symptoms at the menopause in two geographically widely separated samples of British women. Futhermore, in examining the relationship *among* symptoms using cluster analysis technique, they have demonstrated in an alternative way that vasomotor symptoms stand out as being independent from most other physical and psychological symptoms. As in the study by Jaszmann et al. (1969b) the finding that other symptoms occur more frequently in the premenopause than vasomotor ones, peak before they do and, again do so to a much lesser degree, should be noted.

Sharma and Saxena (1981)

This later survey by Sharma and Saxena is of special interest as it is the only one of its kind to be carried out in a third world country. The sample consisted of 405 married women within the age range 40 to 55 years living in the city of Varanasi, in India. The women, who came from all castes, were contacted either through personal contact, women's clubs or public schools. Not surprisingly the sample is biased towards the middle to upper socioeconomic groups. Menopausal status was ascertained by the last menstrual cycle method, and symptoms were elicited by personal interview using the Neugarten and Kraines checklist (see Table 1.2), plus five other symptoms. Only the prevalence of individual symptoms within each menopausal status group was reported.

The overall results were in fact not dissimilar from those obtained by those authors in their survey of women in the United States. Perimenopausal women had higher prevalence rates than premenopausal women for most symptoms, but in only five instances was this greater than 10 per cent. These symptoms were night sweats, weight gain, sleeplessness, feeling blue and mood fluctuations, the largest difference being only 15 per cent for weight gain. Menopausal women also had higher prevalence rates than postmenopausal women of more than 10 per cent only in the case of weight gain, mood fluctuations and palpitations. Thus, there was a clear peaking at the menopause for only two symptoms, out of a total list of 33 symptoms.

Table 3.3

Average Number of Symptoms in Relation to Menopausal Status

	Pre/Post Menopause	Peri-Menopause
Somatic (includes vasomotor)	4.85	5.63
Psychosomatic	3.62	3.96
Psychological	6.10	6.31

Calculated from data in Sharma and Saxena (1981)

To permit a comparison with the findings of Neugarten and Kraines (1965), mean symptom scores for each of the groupings of symptoms used by those authors have been calculated by the present writer on the basis of the data provided in Sharma and Saxena (1981). These are shown in Table 3.3. As can be seen the mean number of symptoms for the Indian women is higher than the American sample within all categories (see Table 3.2). However, the general pattern of results are very similar, with the largest difference between the perimenopausal and non-menopausal Indian women also being for somatic symptoms and the smallest for psychological symptoms. As in previous studies the prevalence rate of symptoms among premenopausal women was considerably high and this may be why so few symptoms showed any clear peaking at the perimenopause. This study is of added interest in having an essentially similar outcome to that of other surveys regarding the relative prevalence of climacteric symptoms at the menopause within an entirely different cultural setting.

Ballinger (1975)

Unlike the preceding six, this survey by Ballinger (1975) is not a study of symptomatology at the menopause as such, but is a study of minor psychiatric illness around that time of life. As a psychiatrist Ballinger's principal interest was to determine the prevalence of psychiatric morbidity at the menopause. The objective was therefore to identify psychiatric cases, and accordingly a standardised instrument designed for this purpose was used. This was the 60 symptom General Hospital Questionnaire (GHQ), a scale developed by Goldberg (1972) to detect possible psychiatric cases, particularly in general practice. Subjects are identified as possible cases if they report more than eleven symptoms. The scale focuses on recent health and is thought mainly to detect mild depressive and neurotic illness. Many of the symptoms in this scale are therefore similar to those used in other surveys of the menopause, hence its relevance to the present discussion. To some extent the use of a standardised instrument could be regarded as a superior method to the ad hoc symptom checklists used in other studies, although it suffers from problems of case definition inherent in psychiatric epidemiology (Wing et al., 1978; Williams et al., 1980). This point is further discussed in section 4.3. Data were gathered by means of a postal questionnaire sent out to women within the age range 40 to 55 years, listed in six general practices in the city of Dundee, Scotland. In addition to the GHQ a brief questionnaire about menstrual cycle and the family situation was included. Menopausal status was determined by the method of McKinlay et al. (1972).

Some 30 per cent of the total number of 539 women responding, were identified as probable psychiatric cases, and of these there was a significantly greater proportion of cases within the perimenopausal group (40 per cent), than the premenopausal (28 per cent) or postmenopausal groups (25 per cent). However, when age was taken into account it was found that although this pattern was repeated within the age ranges 40 to 44 and 50 to 55 years, within the 45 to 49 age range the differences in psychiatric morbidity were less marked. For this age range, which is the one within which most women experience the menopause, the figure for psychiatric morbidity in the premenopausal group was as high as 40 per cent as against 47 per cent in the menopausal group. These figures led Ballinger to conclude that there was a rise in psychiatric morbidity *before* the menopause, which did not persist beyond one year after the cessation of menses. This finding contrasted with vasomotor symptoms, for which there was a highly significant increase only at the perimenopause, which was maintained for up to five years after the end of the menstrual cycle. More psychiatric cases, however, complained of vasomotor symptoms than did non-cases within all groups, regardless as to whether they were pre, peri or postmenopausal.

A number of reservations must be made about this study. The figure of 30 per cent psychiatric morbidity among a general population of women is extremely high, and is almost twice the average prevalence rate for females obtained in other community surveys of psychiatric illness (Goldberg and Huxley, 1980). Furthermore, the finding that within the 45 to 49 years age range almost half of currently menopausal women have a psychiatric illness is difficult to accept. One explanation for this may be that, although designed to detect psychiatric illness, the 60-item version of the GHQ contains one item about hot flushes, and another about sweating. Furthermore, there are at least six items relating to sleep disturbance, a complaint often thought to be due to excessive nocturnal sweating. Clearly then, the high incidence of cases in this group of women, and the increase in cases during the menopause, could be due to the inclusion of these symptoms when applying the relatively low cut off point of eleven symptoms recommended by Goldberg (1972) to identify a case. This could also account for more psychiatric cases having vasomotor symptoms than non-cases.

The psychiatric morbidity rates among menopausal women reported in the survey by Ballinger must therefore be considered spuriously high because of the inclusion of vasomotor symptoms in determining what is a psychiatric case. A similar criticism, couched in more general terms, has been made of this survey by Kaufert and Syrotuik (1981), who have pointed out that as the GHQ contains many physical symptoms 'the somatic and psychosomatic content of the menopausal syndrome may explain the (high) scores made by menopausal women on the GHQ' (p.170). A fuller account of psychiatric illness during the climacteric is given in section 4.3. Nevertheless, what is of interest in this study, given these reservations about the actual levels of minor psychiatric illness among climacteric women, is the finding that any increase in morbidity appears to occur some time *prior* to the actual event of the menopause.

The International Health Foundation Surveys

Two other European surveys which have a bearing on the prevalence of symptoms at the menopause are those which have been carried out under the auspices of the International Health Foundation (IHF), an organisation based in Geneva and founded in 1969 under Swiss law to foster research and education in the medical and related sciences. The surveys, which were carried out in Switzerland and Belgium, were considerably more comprehensive in scope than those previously reviewed, having as their stated objective 'the investigation of the interaction between biological and psychological changes in the ageing women'. Thus, unlike the other surveys reviewed here, which have tended to have been restricted to examining women's symptoms at the climacteric, these surveys in addition to symptoms, examined the influence of the menopause on a wide variety of other social and psychological characteristics such as general adaptation, sexuality, interpersonal relationships, cultural interests and social activities. However, only the findings relating to symptoms will be discussed here, consideration of these other variables being deferred to later chapters.

Methodologically, both surveys also differ from previous ones in that all data were gathered by means of a personal interview of a randomly selected sample of the general population, and not as has often been the case, by postal survey of a non-random sample. In both surveys Jaszmann's criteria for designating menopausal status was used, within the 46 to 55 year age range. The surveys differ from each other in that in the Swiss study, a wider age range of women was sampled, and the method of analysing symptoms in each survey varied in certain important respects.

Considering first the Swiss survey, results are reported (van Keep and Kellerhals, 1974 and 1975; International Health Foundation, 1975) for a random sample of 448 married women, all housewives living in the Zurich area, within the age range 41 to 60 years. Symptoms were assessed by means of a 17 symptom scale, each sympton being rated on a 0 to 3 rating, depending on its frequency of occurrence during the previous month. This yields a total symptom score called a Climacteric Index, which includes vasomotor symptoms, along with other physical and psychological ones. The sample was divided into three age groups — a group of women 'at high risk' to the menopause between 46 and 55 years, a group of younger women between 41 and 45 years and a group of older women between 56 and 60 years. The 46 to 55 years age group was further divided as to whether they were pre, peri or postmenopausal. It was therefore possible in this survey to examine changes in symptoms in relation to chronological as well as 'menstrual' or 'biological' age. These relationships can be seen in Figure 3.4, adapted from van Keep and Kellerhals (1974). This shows what seems to be a gradual increase in symptoms with age, but with a marked spiking at the perimenopause.

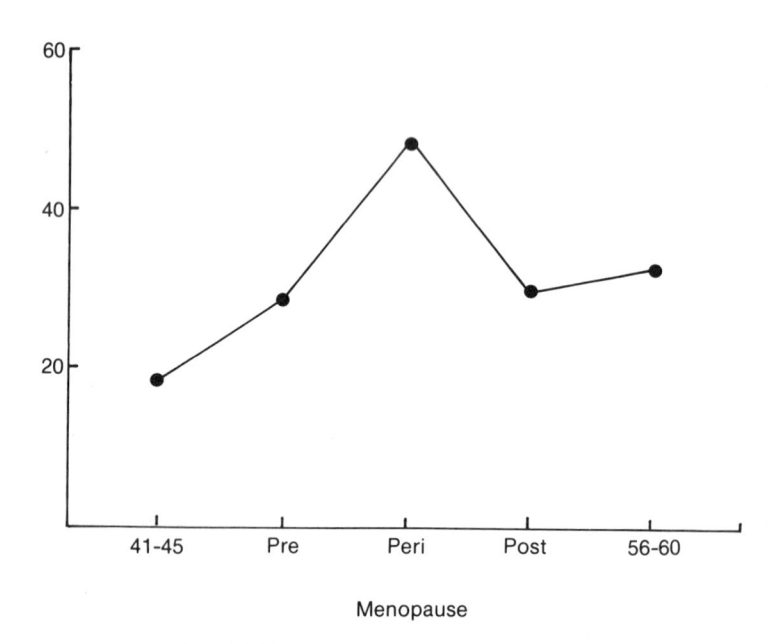

Figure 3.4 Percentages of women with total climacteric index greater than eleven points in relation to age and menopausal status.

(adapted from van Keep and Kellerhals, 1974)

This pattern suggests that at the time of the menopause, an already occurring age related increase in symptoms is simply being exacerbated. There is, however, no way of knowing the extent to which this peaking of symptoms at the menopause is due to an increase in occurrence of vasomotor symptoms, as no separate analysis is presented for these.

Such a distinction was made by Severne in the analysis of the data from the IHF Belgian survey (International Health Foundation, 1977; Severne, 1977 and 1979). Hot flushes and sweats, together with three other 'associated' somatic symptoms, palpitations, paraesthesia and dizziness were combined to form what was called a Circulatory Index, and this was reported separately from a scale consisting of five psychological symptoms — insomnia, nervousness, irritability, headaches and depressive moods, called a Nervosity Index. The separate analyses revealed that these two symptoms indices behaved somewhat differently in relation to menopausal status, although it was not possible, because this survey was restricted to the age range 46 to 55 years, to examine age trends. With regard to the Circulatory Index, this increased markedly, by almost threefold, from the pre to the perimenopausal group, declining only slightly in the postmenopause. The Nervosity Index, while showing a similar pattern, did so to a much lesser degree. These effects can be seen in Figure 3.5 which has been drawn by the present author on the basis of data presented in Severne (1979). It should again be noted that nervous symptoms were more frequent than vasomotor ones during the premenopause.

Comparing these two IHF surveys, it seems likely that the temporary peaking of symptoms at the menopause in the Swiss study was in fact largely due to an increase in vasomotor symptoms. The results of this second survey therefore confirms the differing patterns of change in vasomotor and non-vasomotor in relation to the menopause, and can be compared with the similar pattern obtained by McKinlay and Jefferys (see Figure 3.2). Differences in absolute levels of scores are due to the fact that Severne's scoring system includes a rating of severity, and that the number of symptoms making up each measure varies between the studies. What is important is the similar *temporal pattern* of the measures in relation to menopausal status, confirming the considerably greater degree of association of vasomotor symptoms with the perimenopause. Nevertheless, having said that, the fact that psychological symptoms were more frequent than vasomotor ones during the premenopause and that they showed some peaking at the menopause, would indicate, as suggested above in relation to the IHF Swiss study, that it is an already occurring increase in psychological symptoms which is being further increased at that time. By this is meant that although there is an increase in

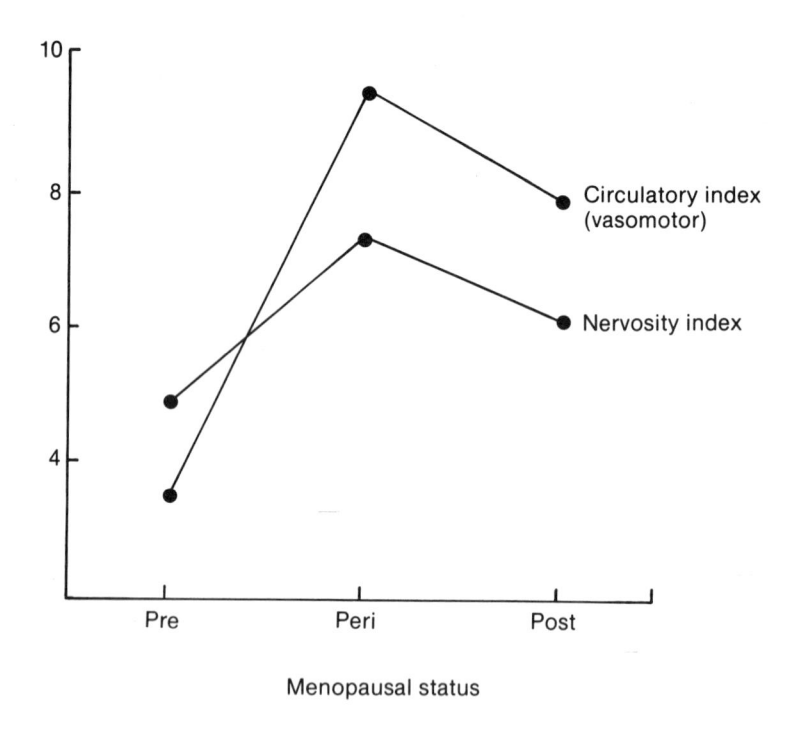

Figure 3.5 Mean scores for two symptom measures in relation to menopausal status. (adapted from Severne, 1979)

symptoms at the time of final menses, this merely represents an *exacerbation* of a more general increase in symptoms which occurs within the climacteric period as a whole.

Greene and Cooke (1980)

Like Severne, these authors also examined the relationship between different types of climacteric symptoms and menopausal status, this time in a sample of urban Scottish women. Subjects were chosen, by systematic sampling from the electoral roll from within the city of Glasgow, Scotland. All information was obtained by means of a personal interview of each subject at her home, the response rate of 85 per cent yielding a total sample of 230 women. For the purpose of this study the climacteric was taken to be the age range 35 to 54 years. Within this age range menopausal status was determined using the criteria of McKinlay et al.

(1972). The main focus of this study was in fact on the relationship between climacteric symptoms and life events, a full account of which is presented in Chapter 8 of this volume. For the moment, however, the relationships found between symptoms, age and menopausal status in this study will be described.

Symptoms were assessed by means of a Climacteric Symptom Rating Scale, consisting of 18 symptoms each rated on a four point scale of severity. These symptoms were subdivided into two main categories, somatic and psychological, on the basis of a previous factor analysis of symptoms presented by women attending a menopausal clinic (Greene, 1976). Vasomotor symptoms (hot flushes and bouts of sweating) were assessed separately, also using a 0 to 3 rating to measure severity. Thus three separate symptom measures were used — one measuring severity of vasomotor symptoms, one the severity of the other physical symptoms and one the severity of psychological symptoms. A full account of this factoral study and the construction of this scale is given in section 7.4, where the Symptom Scale can be found in Table 7.5. There it can be seen that the actual symptoms are not dissimilar from those employed in previous surveys. What differs is that the *separate* and *scaled* measurement of the different types of symptoms has been arrived at on an *empirical* basis.

As a group of younger preclimacteric (25 to 34 years) and a group of older postclimacteric (55 to 64 years) women had been included in the sample, it was possible to examine age trends in symptoms within the 25 to 64 years adult female age range. Inspection of these age trends indicated that mean scores on both the psychological and somatic symptom scales began to rise around the late 30s, reached a peak in the early 40s, declined a little in the late 40s and early 50s and fell off more sharply in the late 50s and early 60s. This elevation in symptoms coincides remarkable closely with the period chosen as the climacteric. These trends are summarised in Figure 3.6 which graphs the mean symptom scores of women between ages 25 to 64 years, grouped in 10-year age bands, for both scales. The climacteric period which, as has been stated earlier, was taken as the age range 35 to 54 years, was therefore subdivided into two periods, one designated early, the other late climacteric.

Figure 3.6 shows a significant peaking for both psychological and somatic symptoms within the *early* climacteric period, which is some time prior to when the majority of women experience the menopause. Vasomotor symptoms on the other hand did not peak until the late climacteric, which is the age range within which the menopause occurs for most women. The relationship between the menopause and the three categories of symptoms was directly examined by calculating average

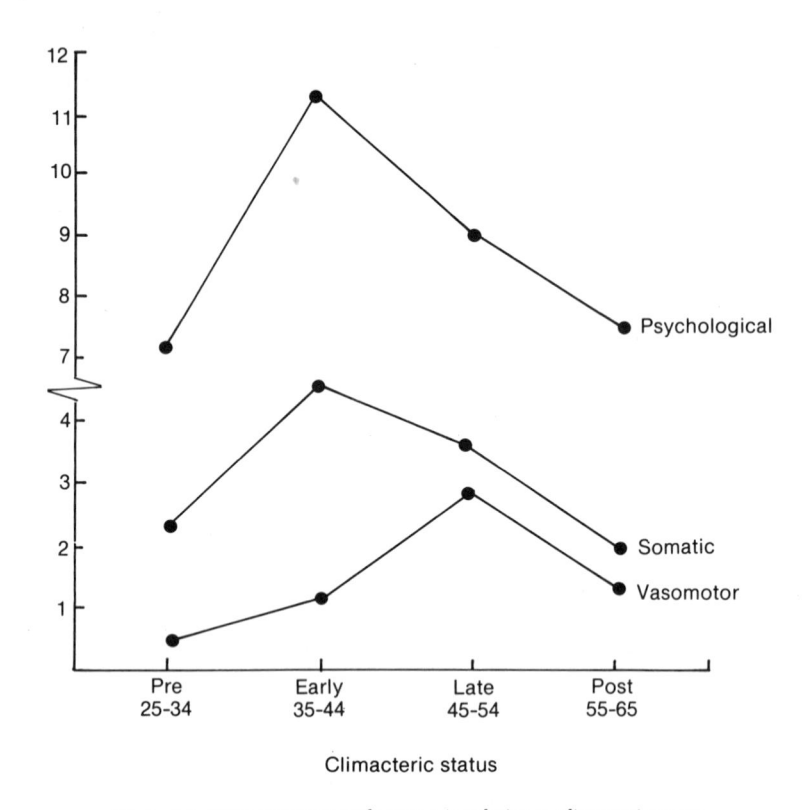

Figure 3.6 Mean symptom scale scores in relation to climacteric status. (from Greene and Cooke, 1980)

scores for pre, peri and postmenopausal women within the climacteric period, that is the 35 to 54 years age range. Although there was a slight increase in both psychological and somatic symptoms at the perimenopause, these increases were not statistically significant. The increase in vasomotor symptoms, on the other hand was considerably greater at the perimenopause and did achieve statistical significance.

Thus, for this sample of Scottish women only vasomotor symptoms bore any close temporal relationship to the time of the menopause. The main increase in other symptoms occurred some time prior to this, in the early climacteric, and was only marginally associated with the menopause. In finding that only the vasomotor measure bore any close association to the menopause, these results are consistent with those of the majority of surveys so far reviewed in this chapter. In addition, the finding that other symptoms tended to peak some time before the menopause would be consistent with those of Jaszmann et al. (1969b) and McKinlay and Jefferys (1974).

Table 3.4 compares the means scores on both scales for the menopausal and postmenopausal climacteric group from the general

Table 3.4

Comparison between Clinical and General Population Groups on Symptom Scales

	General Population Group	Clinical Group
Somatic scale	4.91	7.18
Psychological scale	11.84	19.62

Adapted from Greene (1976)

population sample, with the clinical group on which the scales had originally been developed (Greene, 1976). As can be seen, the symptoms in the clinical group are clearly in excess of those of the normal population, especially in the case of psychological symptoms. This, therefore, confirms the atypical nature of, and the high levels of psychopathology among women attending hormone replacement therapy clinics previously referred to in the introduction to this chapter.

Kaufert and Syrotuik (1981)

As in the study by Greene and Cooke (1980) the symptom measure used in this Canadian survey was also derived from a factor analysis. The sample studied consisted of 148 women living in the city of Winnipeg, and was obtained through a general practice. This is not a randomly collected sample and from the information provided by the authors it is clearly biased towards the upper socioeconomic groups. Data were gathered by means of a postal questionnaire among which were two symptom scales. These two scales consisted of a vasomotor scale of two items (hot flushes and night sweats) and a psychological scale of five items (tiredness, irritability, depression, nervous tension and trouble sleeping). A fuller description of this scale and its construction can be found in section 7.4 of this volume, where the symptoms are shown in Table 7.3. Menopausal status was determined by last menses using Jaszmann's criteria.

The results of this survey were fairly straightforward. The frequency of vasomotor symptoms increased dramatically from the pre to the peri and immediate postmenopause, and continued to increase into the advanced postmenopause (more than five years since last menses). There was little relationship between menopausal status and psychological symptoms. These results are illustrated in Figure 3.7 which shows in fact that psychological symptoms were more frequent at the premenopause than at the perimenopause. Three other physical symptoms which, together with vasomotor symptoms, formed the Circulatory Index in the IHF Belgian survey (Severne, 1979) were also found not to be associated with menopausal status. These were rapid heart beat, dizziness and pins and needles. Although understandably cautious, in view of the size and biased nature of the sample, these authors nevertheless conclude that their

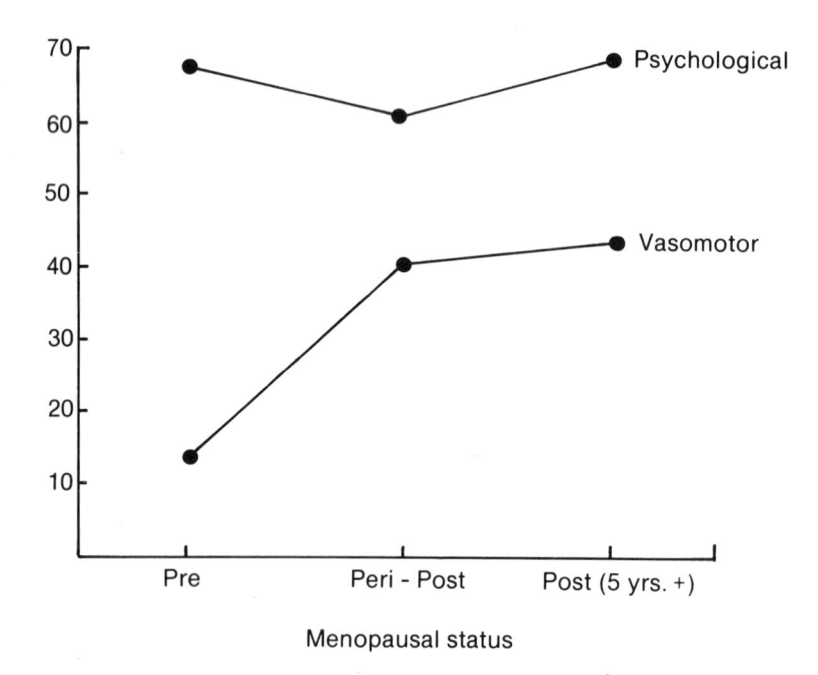

Figure 3.7 Percentages of women reporting symptoms in relation to menopausal status.

(adapted from Kaufert and Syrotuik, 1981)

study 'suggests that there may be no association between menopausal status and levels of psychological morbidity' (p.183). Their results, however, are totally consistent with those of others, and Figure 3.7 can be compared with Figures 3.2 and 3.5. Again differences between surveys in raw figures are due to differences in the measuring instruments. What is more important is the consistently *different* pattern of the two measures (vasomotor and psychological symptoms) in relation to menopausal status.

Mikkelsen and Holte (1982)

This paper consists of a preliminary report from the Norwegian Female Climacteric Project, an as yet uncompleted large scale longitudinal study of the interaction between psychosocial and adverse changes through the climacteric. The results reported here are of a pilot study of 139 women aged between 45 and 56 years, randomly sampled from the official community register of the city of Drammen is south-east Norway. Other results from this study will be discussed in later chapters of this volume. For the moment only the relationships found between symptoms and menopausal status will be described here. All data were collected by means of a postal questionnaire, which among other measures included a checklist of 21 symptoms each rated on a three point scale of severity — never; sometimes; often troubled by the symptom. Symptoms were grouped into six categories made up of a vasomotor category, two categories of psychological and three categories of other physical symptoms. As in the two previous surveys these categories had been formed on the basis of a factor analyses of the 21 symptoms. A fuller account of this factor analysis is also given in Chapter 7, where the symptoms and their categories can be found in Table 7.4. Menopausal status was determined according to time since last menstruation, using a criteria similar to that of McKinlay et al. (1972).

The six symptom categories were then examined in relation to five subgroups of menopausal status, the postmenopausal women being divided into three groups. A one-way analysis of variance was used to determine the significances of differences between subgroups. In brief, it was found that only the vasomotor category of symptoms was significantly related to perimenopausal status, all five other symptom categories failing to distinguish between women of different menopausal status. The authors concluded:

> Excessive sweating, hot flushes and vaginal dryness are the only symptoms that could be included in the concept of the menopausal syndrome.

> The development of the climacteric syndrome may only to some extent be explained in terms of menopausal status. Unexplained variance in the symptoms of the menopausal syndrome may be due to psychosocial factors that require further investigation (p.39).

Thus the findings of this survey of Norwegian women are substantially in agreement with others, using a somewhat more sophisticated method of statistical analysis.

It would appear that where properly constructed scales are used to assess symptoms, as in the preceding three surveys, the tenuous nature of the relationship between psychological symptoms and the event of the menopause becomes all the more clear. This argument is further developed in sections 7.3 and 7.4.

Wood (1979); Bungay, Vessay and McPherson (1980)

Unlike the previous twelve, the final two surveys to be discussed, do not contain comparisons of the prevalence of symptoms among climacteric women of different menopausal status. Rather they report on the prevalence of certain symptoms according to chronological age across samples of the entire female adult population. The argument is that if these symptoms are specific to the menopause, then the prevalence of such symptoms should be higher in the 45 to 54 year age group than in other age groups, that being the age range within which the great majority of women experience the menopause.

The first of these studies, that by Wood (1979), comes from Australia. The data reported were gathered in the course of a major community health and social survey carried out in the north-west suburbs of Melbourne in 1977. The survey was carried out by personal interview of a random cross section of members of the population in their homes. The interviews were structured ones, and conducted by medical students who were specially trained in the technique of collecting accurate information in the home. Symptoms were assessed by means of a 20 item checklist responded to on a present/absent basis. The response rate was 85 per cent and the total sample consisted of 948 women from 20 years upwards. This is a well designed survey and the sample seems to have been representative of the population at large.

Prevalence of symptoms was analysed in terms of chronological age, subdivided into nine five-year age bands. Symptoms were found to follow three types of patterns. They either increased with age, decreased with age, or followed no consistent pattern. Symptoms which increased steadily with age were sleeplessness, joint pains, numbness, palpitations, dizziness and weakness. Those which decreased with age were headaches, skin problems and irritability. Tiredness, fainting, loss of appetite, nervousness, backache, frequency of urination, depression, restlessness, tension and weight gain all showed no association with age. The data was also examined statistically, using a regression analysis, to determine whether or not any symptoms had an unusually high incidence during any of the nine five-year periods, particularly the menopausal periods of 45 to 49 years and 50 to 54 years. None of the symptoms did so within any of the five-year age bands, although inspection of the raw data does show that at least four of the symptoms (headaches, tiredness, tension and nervousness) peaked in the age range 35 to 44 years.

The prevalence of problems at the menopause was also assessed by asking older women an open question as to whether or not they had any problems associated with the menopause. In all, only 7.7 per cent of women reported symptoms other than hot flushes. The authors concluded that no evidence of a menopausal syndrome had been found and that the results were 'consistent with the absence of a multisymptomatic menopausal syndrome as, apart from hot flushes, no other symptom was commonly associated with the menopause' (p.496).

The other survey in which the prevalence of symptoms across a sample of the adult female population was examined in regard to chronological age, was that by Bungay et al. (1980). This survey was carried out in the Oxford Region of England. Symptoms were assessed by means of a postal questionnaire sent out to patients on general practice lists in the Region. In an attempt to improve on earlier work the authors incorporated several special features into their study. Firstly, a sample of men was included to serve, the authors say, as a sort of control group. Secondly, a broad age band of subjects from 30 to 64 years was chosen. Thirdly, the questionnaire was sent out in two parts. The first part consisted of a checklist of 40 different symptoms, each responded to on a present/absent basis, with no reference being made to the menopause either in the questionnaire or covering letter. The second part was sent out six to eight weeks later and was concerned with family, social and gynaecological matters. This procedure was used because, the authors argue, a common defect of previous studies was that, as they were discernible as being concerned with the menopause, responses to symptom checklists were almost certainly biased. A random sample of 1120 women and 510 men were drawn from eight general practitioner practices, stratified to give about equal numbers in each five-year age group in the range 30 to 64 years. Overall response was 70 per cent, the study sample being representative, in social class distribution, of the population from which it was drawn.

In analysing their data the authors calculate rates of positive response to individual symptoms in five-year age groups for each sex separately. Like Wood (1979), the authors justify this method by claiming that the close linking of chronological and menopausal age, enables symptom patterns by chronological age to be interpreted in terms of menopausal age. The data was therefore analysed in terms of symptom prevalence patterns or curves across chronological age. Three such types of patterns were identified by inspection. Firstly, those where male and female curves were parallel, secondly those where male and female curves were not parallel, but the female curve was not related to mean age at menopause and thirdly, those where the male and female curves were not parallel, but the female pattern was related to the age range of the menopause. The last pattern only, was regarded as indicating an association of symptoms with the menopause. Of the 40 symptoms only eleven could be said to follow this pattern in any approximate way. However, of these symptoms only 'the peaks of prevalence of night sweats, day sweats and hot flushing were clearly associated with mean age of menopause, coinciding with it or occurring slightly after it' (p.183). The less impressive peaks of prevalence of a group of mental symptoms (difficulty in concentration, anxiety, loss of confidence, feelings of unworthiness and forgetfulness) were clearly associated with an age just *preceding* menopause. This also held for much smaller peaks of prevalence for symptoms of dizziness, tiredenss and palpitations.

The authors also analysed the data in terms of menopausal status as well, but do not supply the details of the results or how this was done. They do state, however, that this analysis suggested that vasomotor symptoms were more closely related to menopausal status, and mental symptoms to chronological age. Thus, in this age survey there was an elevation of symptoms during the climacteric age range, but only vasomotor symptoms were closely associated with the menopause. Their overall conclusion is that the study 'supports the view that there is a menopausal syndrome, principally affecting vasomotor symptoms' (p.183).

The outcomes of both these age surveys are reasonably consistent with each other, and, despite important differences in methodology, with those of other symptom surveys. Both are agreed that only vasomotor symptoms show any close temporal relationship to the mean age of menopause. As far as other symptoms are concerned, Bungay et al. (1980) find that a number of these increase in prevalence around the age range of the menopause, peaking some time before that event (i.e. during the early climacteric). Wood (1979), while finding no evidence for a peaking of non-vasomotor symptoms at any time during the menopausal age range, did find that a number of symptoms showed a steady increase with age, and that a few also peaked in the early part of the climacteric.

Both surveys are of added interest, since they also demonstrate that many of the symptoms thought to be associated with the menopause and climacteric frequently occur among younger women in the general population, some time before the climacteric. For example, Bungay, et al. (1980) found that within the 30 to 40 years age range, headaches were reported by 25 per cent of women, irritability by around 40 per cent and backache by as many as 45 per cent of women. And this occurs among what seems a fairly representative sample of the normal English female population. The figures obtained by Wood (1979) in Australian women were lower, but still show that such symptoms may run at anywhere

Table 3.5

Summary of the Outcome of General Population Surveys of Symptoms during the Climacteric

Authors	Symptoms Associated with Menopause
Neugarten and Kraines (1965)	Vasomotor, heavy periods, breast pains, weight gain, headaches.
Jaszmann et al. (1969b)	Vasomotor, tingling in extremities, aches in joints and muscles.
Rybo and Westerberg (1971)	Vasomotor only
Thompson et al. (1973)	Vasomotor, palpitations, insomnia.
McKinlay and Jefferys (1974)	Vasomotor, insomnia, weight gain, depression.
Sharma and Saxena (1981)	Vasomotor, weight change, mood fluctuations, insomnia, feeling blue.
Ballinger (1975)	Number of psychiatric cases.
Van Keep and Kellerhals (1974, 1975)	Climacteric index
Severne (1979)	Circulatory (vasomotor) index.
Greene and Cooke (1980)	Vasomotor scale only.
Kaufert and Syrotuik (1981)	Vasomotor scale only.
Mikkelsen and Holte (1982)	Vasomotor scale only.
Wood (1979)	Vasomotor only.
Bungay et al. (1980)	Vasomotor, poor concentration, anxiety, unworthiness, forgetfulness.

between 10 to 30 per cent across the entire female age range. It should be noted that prevalence rates for psychiatric illness in Australian women have also been found to be generally lower than those for women in other countries (Goldberg and Huxley, 1980). It will be recalled that Neugarten and Kraines (1965), whose survey also covered a wide range of women, reported even higher symptom frequencies in younger women. These findings for younger women underline the point made in section 3.1, namely, that the important issue in determining which symptoms are associated with the time of the menopause is the frequency and severity of symptoms at that time *relative* to other times. The outcome of each survey, in that relative sense, is summarised in Table 3.5.

Finally, in this section, and also by way of a summary, Table 3.6 shows the relative prevalence at the menopause of those symptoms, which

Table 3.6

Prevalence of Symptoms among Menopausal Women in Five Surveys

	Neugarten and Kraines (1965)	Sharma and Saxena (1981)	Jaszmann et al. (1969b)	Thompson et al. (1973)	McKinlay and Jefferys (1974)
Hot flushes	68	61	65	74	75
Sweating	32	53	40	31	58
Palpitations	44	75	23	9	38
Dizzy spells	40	74	10	10	30
Headaches	71	86	45	16	38
Insomnia	51	67	35	27	45
Depression	78	68	25	21	55
Rheumatic pains	49	17	45	17	—
Fatigue	88	93	55	21	—
Suffocation	29	44	25	—	—
Numbness and tingling	37	69	22	—	—
Irritable	92	67	35	—	—
Weight gain	61	70	—	—	50

have been most commonly asked about in surveys. These come from the five surveys in which the prevalence of individual symptoms have been reported, as opposed to total scores. As can be seen the only symptom about which there is any consensus as to their prevalence rates are hot flushes. The proportion of women reporting hot flushes averages out at about two-thirds, and sweating at just over one-third. It is worth noting that these averages are closest to the actual figures of Jaszmann et al. (1969b) whose sample was by far the most representative of all five surveys. On the basis of probability this is exactly what one would expect. For all other symptoms there is a wide variation in prevalence. Some of these variations in other symptoms may be due to 'real' differences between the populations studied. For example, the very high frequency of somatic symptoms among Indian women in the survey by Sharma and Saxena (1981) could be due to cultural factors, a theme we shall return to in section 6.2. Some of the variation, however, could be due to differences between studies in methodology, a theme we shall be returning to in Chapter 7.

3.3. SUMMARY AND CONCLUSION

Despite the wide variation in methods employed in these fourteen surveys, the striking feature of their outcome is their remarkable agreement regarding the central issues. That is, the issues of the prevalence of different symptoms at the menopause and the existence of a multisymptom menopausal syndrome. The following points can be made on the basis of the foregoing review.

1. In all fourteen surveys the only symptoms which consistently stand out as being closely associated with the menopause are the vasomotor ones. These symptoms rise sharply in prevalence close to the time of final menses and may continue to do so for one or two years into the postmenopause, thereafter declining. In no survey do any other symptoms, or types of symptoms, follow the same consistent and marked temporal relationship to the menopause.
2. While there is a unanimous consensus that hot flushes and sweating are closely associated with the time of the menopause, there is less consistent agreement as to whether any other symptoms bear any relationship to the menopause. Indeed in

five surveys no symptoms or types of symptoms, other than vasomotor ones, were found to increase significantly at that time. In contrast, seven of the remaining nine surveys do provide evidence that in addition to vasomotor symptoms a few others do increase in prevalence at the menopause, but there is little consensus as to which particular symptoms these are (see Table 3.5).
3. Where other symptoms have been found to increase in prevalence at the time of final menses, the magnitude of this increase is invariably less than that of vasomotor symptoms, and in addition, many are found to be fairly common *prior* to the perimenopause, in comparison with vasomotor symptoms. To take one example, McKinlay and Jefferys (1974) found the rate of depression in premenopausal women to be 39 per cent, rising to 55 per cent at the perimenopause. The equivalent figures for hot flushes were 18 per cent and 75 per cent respectively. Figure 3.5 shows a similar pattern for composite symptom scales.
4. Futhermore, many of the non-vasomotor symptoms which show no increase whatsoever at the menopause are also fairly common during the premenopause, and indeed many of these peak at that time and may be declining while vasomotor symptoms are increasing in prevalence (see Figures 3.1, 3.2, 3.6 and 3.7). Surveys examining age trends show similar patterns for some symptoms.
5. Finally, the only symptoms about which there seems to be any consensus regarding their actual prevalence rate at the menopause are the vasomotor ones, there being considerable variation in regard to the prevalence of other 'core' symptoms at that time (see Table 3.6).

Conclusion

For the foregoing reasons it can be concluded that there is little empirical support for the existence of a multisymptom syndrome associated with the menopause, among the general population of climacteric women. Once again it is only those symptoms, which there is good reason to suppose are of hormonal origin, which show any marked and consistent temporal relationship to that event. Where other symptoms have been found to increase around the time of the menopause, there is little consensus as to which symptoms these are, or their prevalence rates. Their increase is invariably much less than that of vasomotor ones, they are found to be relatively numerous among premenopausal women, and some tend to increase and peak in prevalence some time prior to the actual menopause. Thus, what we have chosen to call non-specific symptoms are already occurring at fairly high levels among women in early middle age, perhaps as part of a more general climacteric or age related increase. At the time of the menopause some of these symptoms may be *exacerbated*, either for symbolic reasons, or for reason of 'physiological instability', due to a critical stage having been reached in the atrophy of the ovaries. Vasomotor symptoms, on the other hand, are comparatively infrequent prior to the menopause, but increase dramatically with the onset of that event, and may continue to do so for some time into the immediate postmenopause.

Therefore, although there is little evidence from general population surveys to support the notion of a multisymptom menopausal syndrome per se, there are indications that there is indeed an increase in the prevalence of non-specific symptoms throughout the age range of the climacteric, probably beginning in the earlier part. This perhaps justifies the nomenclature 'climacteric syndrome', the aetiology of which, as stated at the end of Chapter 1, is subject to further empirical investigation. For the remainder of this volume, therefore, the phrases climacteric syndrome or climacteric symptoms will refer to those non-specific symptoms, experienced by women at that time of life, which cannot be attributed to a recognised medical, psychiatric or psychological condition.

4

Other Aspects of Women's Functioning During the Climacteric

So far in this volume we have confined ourselves to an examination of the association between the climacteric period and the symptomatology presented by women at that time. That is, the reporting of symptoms, and in particular psychological ones, has been seen as an important measure of adverse reaction. However, it is often thought that during the climacteric in general, and at the menopause in particular, more widespread psychological changes occur and that indeed the increase in non-specific symptoms may merely be an expression of other more specific problems and changes. In this chapter we will therefore consider the empirical evidence regarding what changes may occur in other aspects of women's social and psychological functioning at that time. Unfortunately, there are few empirical studies in this area. The only studies in which such characteristics have been examined in any comprehensive way have been the two International Health Foundation surveys, already described in the preceding chapter. This chapter will therefore begin with an account of the findings from these two surveys relevant to this issue. Thereafter, evidence of changes, during the climacteric, in another important aspect of female functioning, namely sexual behaviour, will be reviewed. The chapter will then conclude with an examination of the psychiatric literature to determine the extent to which climacteric symptomatology may be accounted for by the occurrence of formal psychiatric illness, peculiar or otherwise, to that time of life. In this chapter, therefore, psychological and social changes which occur among women during the climacteric are being regarded, like symptoms in the previous chapter, as dependent variables.

4.1 THE INTERNATIONAL HEALTH FOUNDATION STUDIES

As noted in section 3.2, where the relationship between menopausal status and symptoms was discussed, both IHF studies were considerably more comprehensive in scope than other surveys reviewed therein, in going beyond the consideration of symptoms alone, to include an examination of changes in a variety of other psychological and social characteristics of women during the climacteric. Indeed these studies are the only ones published to date which aimed to obtain a broad picture of the changes which occur in women's overall self evaluation, her social activities, interests and interpersonal relationships at that time, and as such their findings are worth special and detailed consideration.

The IHF Swiss Study

In the report on the Swiss study (International Health Foundation, 1975) these various characteristics were grouped into four broad categories — Subjective Adaptation, Role Identity, Immediate Family Relations and Wider Social Relations. The details and content of these categories are listed in Table 4.1. Questionnaires were devised by the research team to assess these characteristics in the form of self ratings. It will be recalled

Table 4.1
Psychological and Social Characteristics Examined in the International Health Foundation Surveys

Characteristic	Description
Subjective Adaptation	Satisfaction with daily life, health, physical appearance and daily tasks; view of future.
Role identity	Dependency on others; identification with traditional female, maternal and sexual roles.
Immediate Family Relations	Marital and sexual relations; emotional relationship with children; family conflicts.
Wider Social Relations	Cultural activities; relational integration (social contacts); normative integration (social values).

that it had been possible in section 3.2, because of the relatively wide age range investigated, to examine symptoms in relation to both age and menopausal status. Changes in the above characteristics will now also be summarised in relation to these two factors.

Subjective Adaptation. The overall trend was for this to decrease fairly rapidly with age, with a marked dip at the perimenopause. All the items of this measure behaved in much the same way.

Role Identity. These items all behaved differently in respect to age and menopausal status. Dependency on others tended to increase with age but showed no relation to menopausal status. Identification with the maternal role showed no change with age, but decreased slightly during the perimenopause. Positive evaluation of the sex role showed a slight overall decline with age, a decline which like Subjective Adaptation was also exacerbated at the menopause.

Immediate Family Relations. Sexual relations, both frequency and pleasure therefrom, also declined with age but were not influenced by menopausal status. These findings are further discussed in section 4.2 of this chapter. The perimenopause was, however, associated with a slight increase in marital and family disharmony leading the authors to comment that 'the familial climate is disturbed around the menopause but not as much as many suppose' (IHF, 1975, p.35).

Wider Social Relations. The number of cultural activities engaged in, current social involvement and normative integration, a measure of how much a woman adheres to current social values, all gradually declined with age, declines which in all cases were not greatly affected at the menopause.

Virtually all these social and psychological characteristics therefore declined at varying rates with age, any change at the time of the menopause being either an exacerbation of this age related decline, or possibly in some instances the initiation of one. Examples of these effects on four measures, one taken from each of the categories listed in Table 4.1, are illustrated in Figures 4.1 and 4.2. In Figure 4.1 two measures are

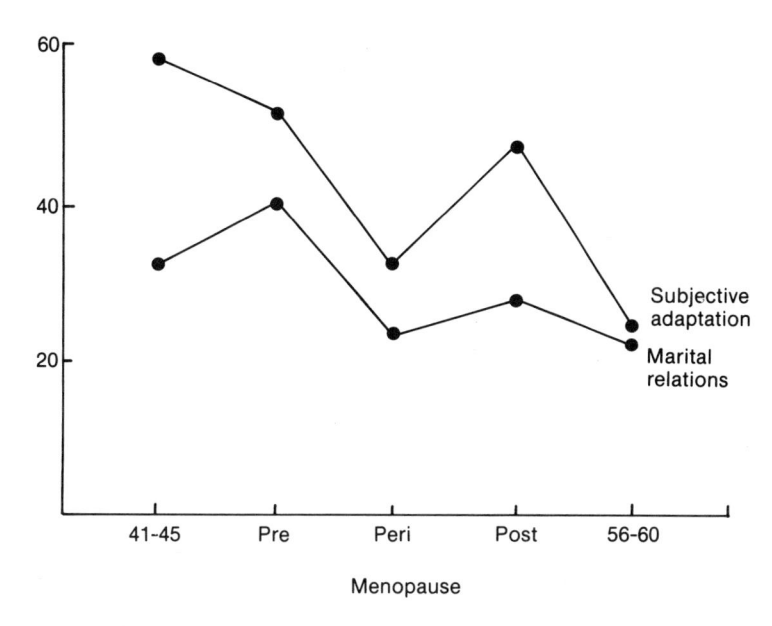

Figure 4.1 Percentage of women showing good subjective adaptation and good relations with spouse in relation to age and menopausal status.
(adapted from van Keep and Kellerhals, 1974 and IHF, 1975)

seen to decline with age and to dip temporarily at the menopause, whereas in Figure 4.2 there is a much less marked association with age and no dip at final menses. In the latter cases the age decline could be regarded as begining around the time of final menses. Both the other items relating to Wider Social Relations, (cultural activities and relational integration) followed a similar pattern to normative integration.

Thus, as with many symptoms (see conclusion, section 3.3), any change at the time of the menopause tends to be an exacerbation of an already occurring age effect. A further important point is that this

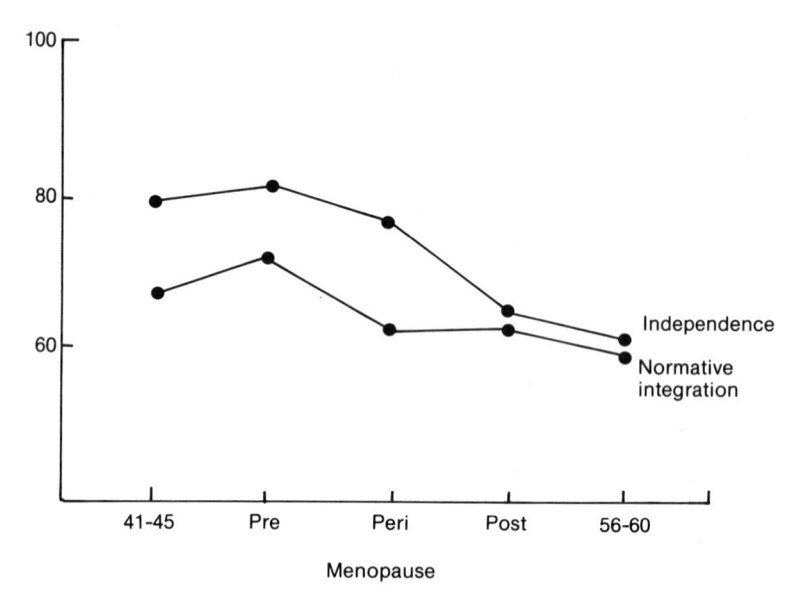

Figure 4.2 Percentages of women showing high independence and good normative integration in relation to age and menopausal status.
(adapted from IHF, 1975)

exacerbation effect, or more accurately, acceleration effect, tends to be confined more to personal physical and psychological self evaluation, that is Subjective Adaptation, and to a lesser degree Immediate Family Relations, rather than related to attitudes, interests and social relationships within a wider setting.

The IHF Belgian Study

Changes at the menopause in these various psychological and social characteristics were also examined in the other IHF survey, that carried out in Belgium by Severne (1979). However, as the age range of the women in that survey was a narrower one, between 45 to 54 years, only changes in relation to menopausal status, could be examined. By and large the results seem to be very similar to those obtained in the Swiss survey. Figure 4.3, adapted from Severne (1979), illustrates the association between menopausal status and two of the measures, confirming that as in the Swiss study, the decline at the menopause in the more personal Subjective Adaptation is greater than that for the more general types of characteristics included under Wider Social Relations.

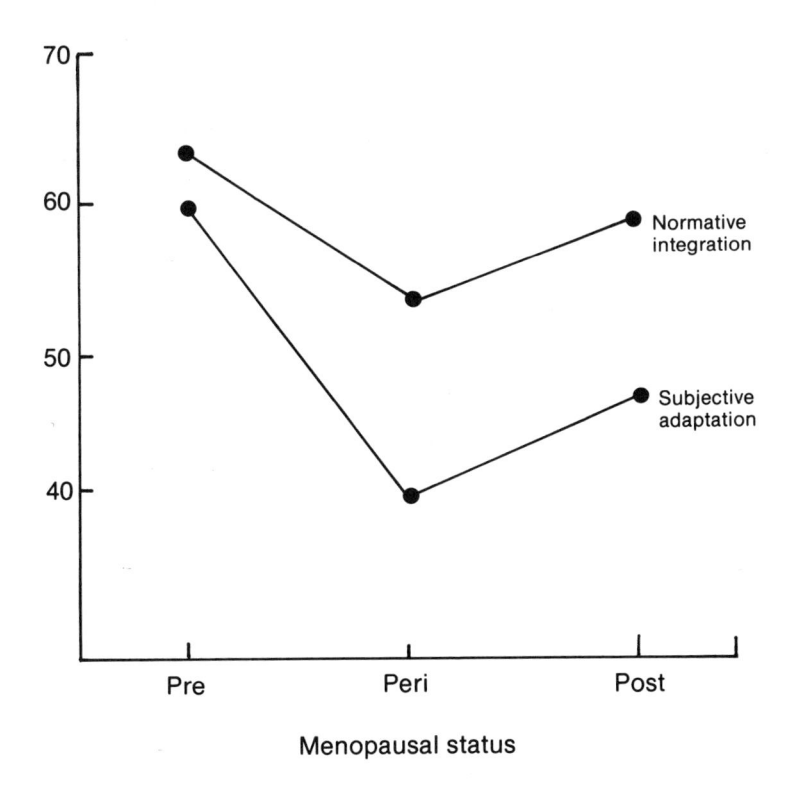

Figure 4.3 Percentages of women showing good subjective adaptation and normative integration in relation to menopausal status.
(adapted from Severne, 1979)

This would lend further support to the suggestion made above, that at the menopause there is an acceleration in the rate of decline of those functions which decline most rapidly with age.

Despite their findings, the authors of the Swiss survey in the discussion section of their report (IHF, 1975) frequently use the term 'menopausal crisis' and it is difficult to concur wholly with their final conclusion, namely that 'it is clear that for many women the menopause is a period of disorientation, physical problems and psychological imbalance' (p.49). The impact of the menopause per se on most of the psychological and social characteristics of middle aged women in this survey appears to be relatively benign, certainly in comparison with that of chronological age. Severne, on the other hand, in her discussion of the Belgian study plays down the impact of the menopause and concludes that 'the actual physical event of the menopause appears in the opinion of the women themselves of rather limited importance. The same holds for the emotional changes as reflected in their relations with the immediate human environment and in their attitudes towards self and social values' (p.119). This seems a more balanced and acceptable judgement, and one which could equally apply to both IHF surveys.

4.2. SEXUAL FUNCTIONING DURING THE CLIMACTERIC

The time of the climacteric is often linked in people's minds with a decrease in a woman's sexual interest and responsiveness. This is not surprising in view of the now well established hormonal basis of sexual behaviour and some forms of sexual dysfunction (Bancroft, 1978 and 1980). In addition, it would appear that a substantial number of women presenting at hormone replacement clinics have such complaints. For example, Studd and Parsons (1977) claim that nearly half of patients attending a hospital based menopause clinic gave sexual symptoms among their three main complaints. Women attending such clinics however, are unlikely to be representative of the female population in general and may include women with longstanding psychosexual problems. As noted in the introduction to Chapter 3, very high levels of psychopathology have been recorded, in a number of different countries of the world, among women attending gynaecological clinics. Figures of sexual complaints from clinical populations are, therefore, not likely to reflect their prevalence in the normal population of climacteric females. For this reason estimates of psychosexual difficulties, as with other problems at the climacteric, must be derived from studies of general populations.

General Population Studies

In only three of the fourteen surveys discussed in Chapter 3 was information relating to sexual behaviour at the menopause obtained. These were the age survey by Bungay et al. (1980) in England, the survey by Ballinger (1975) of psychiatric morbidity in Scottish women, and the IHF Swiss survey by van Keep and Kellerhals (1975). In the first study both 'difficulty with intercourse' and 'loss of interest in sexual relations' were included in the 40 item checklist. Among women, difficulty with intercourse showed a steady and gradual increase from the thirties through to the sixties. Loss of interest in sexual relations followed a similar pattern, but with a slight temporary increase in prevalence of about 5 per cent during the mid forties. These age trends are illustrated in Figure 4.4. Neither of these symptoms showed any particular tendency therefore, to increase at age of menopause. Nor did Ballinger (1976) find

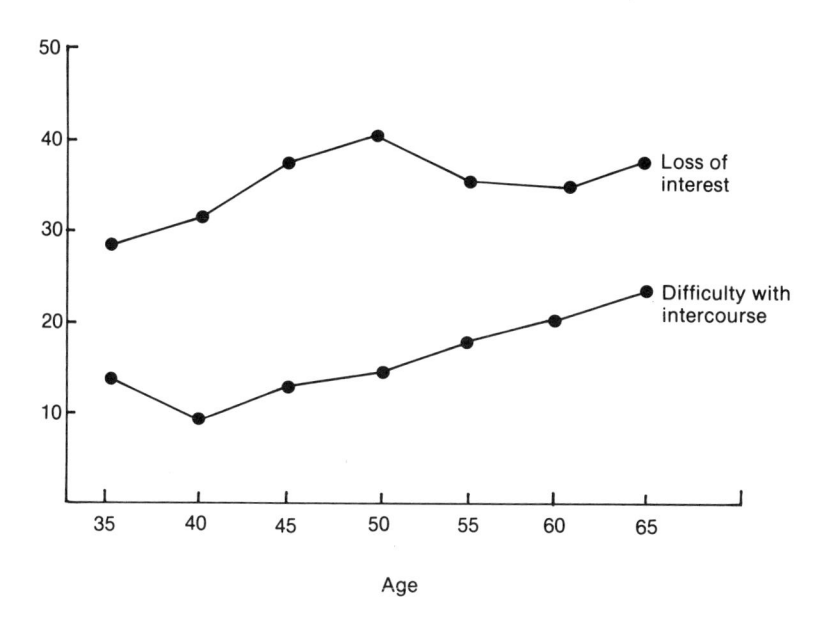

Figure 4.4 Percentages of women reporting sexual problems in relation to age. (adapted from Bungay et al., 1980)

evidence of any appreciable change in libido at or after the menopause in 'psychiatric cases'. Many of these women certainly expressed dissatisfaction with their sexual relations, but as many as 25 per cent stated that they had *never* enjoyed sexual relations. Moreover, these women were more likely to express dissatisfaction with their marital relations as a whole. Ballinger thought that 'both these complaints may be related to the problem that many neurotic patients have with interpersonal relationships in general' (p.1185). In the IHF Swiss study both frequency of sexual intercourse and pleasure therefrom, remained relatively high at the menopause but both decreased sharply in the older 56 to 60 years age range. This effect is illustrated for sexual pleasure in

Figure 4.5. In none of these surveys therefore was there any particular association between the menopause and sexual behaviour, rather any such changes either tended to be age related or else the problem may have been a pre-existing one.

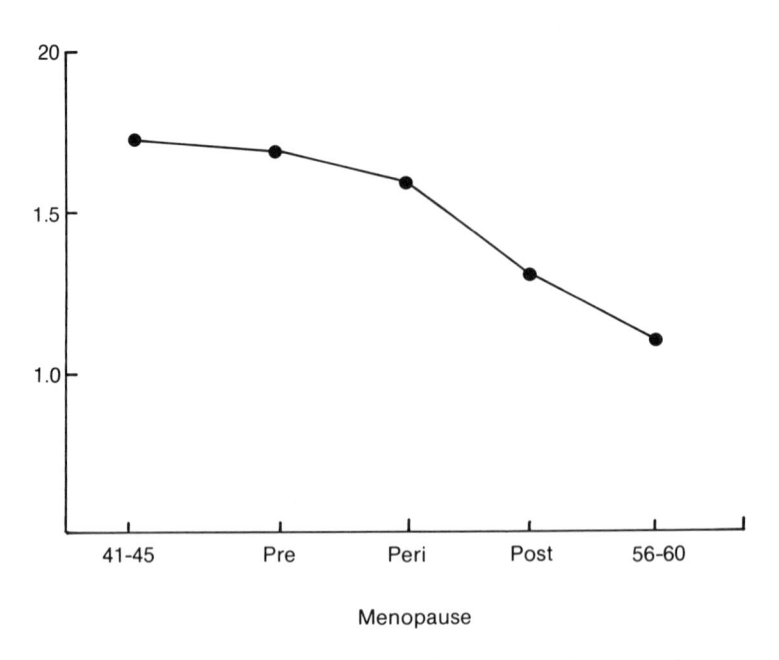

Figure 4.5 Index of sexual pleasure in relation to age and menopausal status. (adapted from IHF, 1975)

These age related declines in sexual functioning are consistent with the observations made by Kinsey and his colleagues in their seminal work carried out in the United States in the early fifties. These researchers had reported a steady decline over the entire age span in the sexual activity of married women (Kinsey et al., 1953) over the years from 20 to 60 years, there being no tendency for there to be any deviation in this steady fall during the menopausal years. Furthermore, when women did report a decline in sexual response following the menopause, this was seen by the authors not as a consequence of the menopause, but as due to other factors operating in the women's lives at that time, or to their use of the menopause as an excuse for giving up a sexual relationship which had never been particularly rewarding. A similar gradual and steady decline in all aspects of sexual functioning was demonstrated by Christenson and

Gagnon (1965) in a later general population study of American women in their post fifties. These authors in addition found that the only factors associated with this age decline was religious devoutness and age of husband.

This association of decreasing sexual interest and activity with age, was also reported in two later general population studies, in both of which the role of the menopause in this decline was specifically examined. Pfeiffer and Davis (1972) and Pfeiffer et al. (1972), in a survey of sexual behaviour in a group of men and women between the ages of 45 to 69 years, found the overall pattern to be one of declining sexual interest and activity with age. Differences were observed between men and women in regard to all indicators of sexual behaviours, with women generally reporting more reduced sexual functioning than men. However, when the effect of age was excluded statistically by means of a stepwise multiple regression, being postmenopausal made a small but significant independent contribution to sexual dysfunction, but age still proved to be the most important factor. That is, although the decline with age proved to be the most prominent pattern, there was a tendency for this decline to be slightly exacerbated at the menopause. These authors however, also found that this decline was greater among women who had not derived much enjoyment from sexual experiences in their earlier years.

Evidence for a stronger effect of menopausal status per se on decline in sexual functioning comes from a survey by Hallstrom (1973, 1977) carried out in Sweden. This is one of the most comprehensive surveys of sexuality among women at the climacteric to have been carried out to date. Eight hundred climacteric women were sampled from three age strata, 46, 50 and 54 years, together with a 38 year old preclimacteric group. Again the main trend was for all aspects of sexual behaviour — sexual interest, capacity for orgasm and coital frequency — to decline with age. These trends are summarised in Figure 4.6. Being postmenopausal per se was also associated with a decline in all aspects of sexual functioning, and this held even when women were matched for age. These results therefore indicate the presence of an impairment in sexual function during the climacteric, independent from the effect of age alone. However, several other factors such as, social class, mental health status, psychosocial stress and an unhappy marital situation were also associated with decreased sexual functioning at the climacteric. The last finding concurs with that of an earlier study by Clark and Wallin (1965) who found that marital relations described as 'negative' were associated with decreased sexual responsiveness among women in the later years of marriage. Quoting from Masters and Johnson (1966), Hallstrom concludes that 'it has become increasingly evident that the psyche plays a

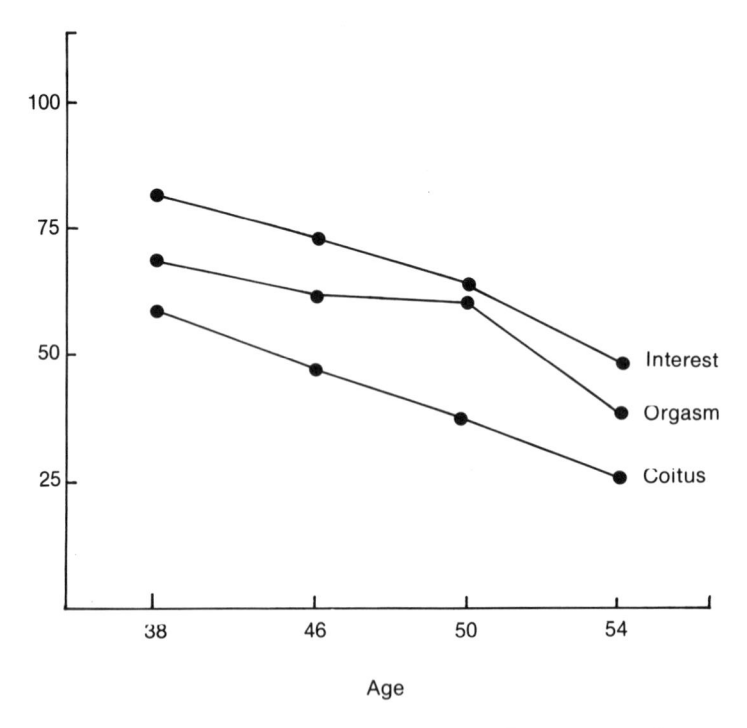

Figure 4.6 Sexual interest (percent strong – moderate), capacity for orgasm (percent always – occasionally) and frequency of coitus (number per year) in relation to age.

(adapted from Hallstrom, 1977)

part at least equal to, if not greater than, that of an imbalanced endocrine system in determining the sex drive of women in the postmenopausal period of their lives' (p.237). Hallstrom also noted that dyspareunia, a symptom associated with atrophic vaginitis, accounted for some loss of sexual interest, but only in about 8 per cent of women, although this figure may be higher among women attending menopause clinics. No relation was found, however, between impairment of sexual interest and total oestrogen output in a subsample of 146 postmenopausal women.

Further evidence of an accentuation at the time of the menopause of the age related decline in sexual functioning, comes from a study of a clinical population of Italian women by Bottiglioni and De Aloysio (1982). These authors examined various aspects of sexual behaviour (absence of intercourse, sexual satisfaction, orgasmic and coital frequency, sexual drive) in a group of 756 Italian women between 40 to 65 years, attending a menopause clinic in Bologna. As usual, age was found to play a predominant role in declining sexual activity, there being a marked fall off in all the above aspects of sexual activity in the fourth and fifth decades. When age was controlled for, the premenopause was found to be associated with a slightly lesser decline in sexual satisfaction, orgasmic response and sexual drive. The authors concluded that as a woman's age advances there is a progressive decline in sexuality and that the menopause accentuates this decline. However, as all these women were attending a menopause clinic, it is possible that a number of the menopausal women were doing so because of sexual difficulties, thereby increasing the incidence of such problems in that group.

Like Hallstrom (1973), van Keep and Kellerhals (1975) in the IHF survey of Swiss women, also observed an association between social class and sexual behaviour among climacteric women, finding that both frequency of and pleasure from sexual intercourse was lower in women of low socioeconomic status at all ages and within all menopausal status groups than in those of high socioeconomic status. Although not a study of the effect of age or menopausal status on sexual behaviour as such, a survey by Garde and Lunde (1980a; 1980b) in Denmark, is of some relevance to these findings. These authors report on a detailed and comprehensive survey of different aspects, both past and present, of sexuality in relation to social class, in a random sample of 225, 40 year old Danish women. As far as current sexual activity was concerned women of lower social class less frequently experienced orgasm and had a considerably higher frequency of sexual problems (48 per cent) than those of higher socioeconomic status (9 per cent). In addition, women of lower social class had a poor knowledge, understanding and acceptance of sexual matters. These results would be consistent with Hallstrom's conclusion that at least some of the decline in sexual functioning during the early climacteric years is associated with psychological and social factors.

Thus the evidence for a decline in sexual functioning associated with the climacteric, and the menopause specifically, is equivocal. However, even if there should be such a change, it would appear to be merely an acceleration of an already ongoing age related decline, as has been seen in the previous section of this chapter, in regard to some other social and psychological characteristics. In addition, it would appear that any such decline may be accentuated by a number of other factors, such as sexual habits and interest in earlier years, social class, mental health, marital satisfaction and poor interpersonal relationships. The question of the role of hormonal changes in this decline of sexual interest and performance is still, however, an open one and cannot as yet be resolved by existing studies of the general population of women.

Libido Following Oophorectomy

In this context, studies of libido in women following surgical menopause, where the ovaries have been removed by operation, might help unravel the confounding effects of age and the menopause on sexual functioning, as such women tend to be younger than those experiencing the natural menopause. Estimates of diminished sexual functioning following hysterectomy and/or oophorectomy of 10, 15, 18 and 38 per cent have been reported by Huffman (1950), Dodds et al. (1961), Patterson and Craig (1963) and Richards (1973) respectively. None of these reports however, throw much light on its aetiology.

More recently, Chakravarti et al. (1977) have reported a loss of libido of as high as 46 per cent among oophorectomised women. These women were followed up from between one and 31 years after surgery, and for almost half, it had been more than eight years since their operation. Furthermore, their ages ranged from 32 to 71 years. These authors claim that this study 'reveals the severity of vasomotor, sexual and depressive symptoms following oophorectomy, and that oestrogen therapy had been rarely prescribed to correct this debilitating climacteric syndrome' (p.774). This is a surprising conclusion, since to attribute loss of libido to the loss of ovaries in such a group of women seems to be highly dubious. However, it does serve to highlight the quality of some of the supposedly 'scientific' medical research in this area.

Utian (1975), on the other hand, in a well designed study, investigated sexual functioning in a mixed group of pre and postmenopausal women *shortly* after hysterectomy, during which some women had their ovaries removed and others not. About one-third of these women complained for up to two years postoperatively, of decreased or absent libido, regardless of menopausal status and regardless of whether or not the ovaries had been removed. These results are summarised in Table 4.2. Thus, loss of libido did not appear to depend on oestrogen deprivation. Although any conclusion regarding the cause of this decreased libido was, according to the author, beyond the scope of the study, Utian does conclude that 'a psychological response to the operation of hysterectomy per se cannot be excluded' (p.4).

Dennerstein et al. (1977) report a similar study of 89 patients, all of whom had undergone both hysterectomy and oophorectomy. Women were asked about various aspects of their sexual relations postoperatively, including sexual desire and enjoyment, frequency of orgasm, dyspareunia, etc. Using an overall rating of sexual dysfunction approximately one-third of the women fell into the three categories of deteriorated, improved and no change, which is consistent with the

Table 4.2

Percentage of Women Complaining of Loss of Libido Postoperatively

Libido	Hysterectomy + Oophorectomy		Hysterectomy alone	
	6 months	2 years	6 months	2 years
Normal	61	61	75	67
Decreased	39	39	25	33
	100	100	100	100

Adapted from Utlan (1975)

finding of Utian (1975). Women had also been asked about any preoperative anxieties they might have had. It was found that women who had had preoperative anxieties about possible deterioration of sexual functioning were those for whom there had been a greater subsequent deterioration in sexual behaviour, especially loss of desire and dyspareunia. These results are summarised in Table 4.3. These authors conclude 'that psychological factors, particularly an expectation that the operation will adversely affect sexual relations, are responsible for the deterioration in sexual relations which follows this operation' (p.96).

Table 4.3

The Relation between Sexual
Anxieties and Postoperative Sexual Response

Overall Sexual Outcome	Sexual Anxieties	
	Absent	Present
Improved	40	26
Same	36	21
Worse	23	53
	100	100

Adapted from Dennerstein et al. (1977)

It is worth noting here that, some three decades ago, Kinsey et al. (1953) also presented data on 123 oophorectomised women and 173 women who had gone through a natural menopause. In both groups, just more than half experienced a decline in sexual activity, most of the rest were unchanged, and indeed a small number became more responsive. A similar number of non-menopausal women of the same age, experienced a similar decline in sexual activity, thereby indicating that change in sexual activity could not be attributed to loss of ovarian function.

Libido and Oestrogen Therapy

So far, it would seem that when the menopause is found to be associated with decline in sexual interest, any such change around that time is likely to be age related or have psychological or social origins. From the point of view of establishing a hormonal basis to the loss of interest, the effects of oestrogen on reduced libido is clearly of relevance. Neither Utian (1975) nor Dennerstein et al. (1977), in the studies of hysterectomised and oophorectomised women, just referred to, found oestrogen therapy to be of any benefit in the treatment of decreased or absent libido following the operation.

In three of the controlled clinical trials previously discussed in section 2.3, the effect of oestrogen replacement on sexual dysfunction had also been reported. Campbell and Whitehead (1977), in their comprehensive trials of women experiencing a natural menopause, found neither placebo nor oestrogen to have any significant effect on libido as reflected in coital satisfaction, frequency of coitus and orgasm, despite a significantly greater improvement of vaginal dryness after oestrogen. Similarly, Paterson (1982) found placebo and oestrogen to have no effect whatsoever on two symptoms of sexual dysfunction, loss of sexual interest and difficulty with intercourse. A 'certain impairment' in sexual functioning was noted in the clinical trial by Fedor-Freybergh (1977) in the placebo group, but the author also noted that the number of patients was too small to allow definite conclusions to be drawn regarding the beneficial effects of oestrogen on libido. However, as has been pointed out in section 2.3 no reference is made in this last study as to the extent vasomotor symptoms were alleviated by oestrogen, and therefore to what extent any improvement in other areas, including sexual functioning, could have been secondary to this. In other words, as Townsend et al. (1980) have argued, a domino effect could operate in the case of sexual dysfunction, as it does for other symptoms and complaints.

That this may be the case was clearly demonstrated in an uncontrolled study by Maoz and Durst (1980). These authors found that the majority of a group of postmenopausal women reported no change in sexual functioning following oestrogen therapy. Among the few women who did report such improvement 'the most important finding was that none of the women showed a positive change in sexual activity *without* the abatement of hot flushes' (p.332, present author's italics).

The only controlled trial in which a clear beneficial effect of oestrogen on sexual dysfunction has been reported is that by Dennerstein et al. (1980) — a finding which is contrary to that reported in their early 1977 paper. This study has been previously described and criticised in section 2.3 regarding the authors' claim of a similar beneficial effect of oestrogen on mood. In effect the criticisms to be made here of the sexual aspects of this research are not dissimilar. Compared with a placebo there were improvements on interviewer ratings of patients' sexual desire and enjoyment, following three months oestrogen therapy. There was also a reported increase in orgasmic frequency. As in the other paper the authors went on to examine the extent to which improved sexual functioning could be a result of relief of vasomotor symptoms, using analysis of co-variance, but this was done *only* with regard to orgasmic frequency. As the improvement in orgasmic frequency, although reduced, remained significant after the effect of hot flushes had been co-varied out, the authors concluded that 'this finding suggests a direct influence of hormones on certain aspects of sexuality' (p.321). A number of critical points can be made. The finding of an increase in orgasmic frequency as a result of oestrogen therapy is only one positive finding among a number of negative ones. No improvement was noted in frequency of intercourse, nor in any of *fifteen* ratings of sexual response made by women themselves using visual analogue scales. Furthermore, sexual desire was found to correlate with several measures of mood, including general feelings of wellbeing, with which the correlations rose to as high as 0.89. Any reported improvement in sexual desire, therefore, could have been due to improvement in mood, which in turn could have been due, as has been argued before (section 2.3), to relief from hot flushes. Although this is a well designed study the authors' interpretation of their results is questionable, and they have not convincingly demonstrated any direct effect of oestrogen on sexuality.

One gynaecologist, who with his colleagues has repeatedly claimed remarkable improvements among menopausal women of sexual dysfunction as a result of hormone replacement therapy, is Studd (Studd et al., 1977a; Studd et al., 1977b; Studd and Parsons, 1977). These claims are based on the use of hormone treatment with a series of patients attending a menopause clinic in London. It is not a controlled trial in any sense. Initially, it was found that both oral and subcutaneously implanted oestradiol produced a marked improvement in dyspareunia, but had little effect on libido. Patients complaining of the latter were then treated with a combined hormone implant of oestradiol and testosterone. These authors write that 'a significant improvement in libido was noted in 80 per cent of these patients who found that their sexual response was better or as good as before the climacteric' (Studd et al., 1977b, p.315). This occurred despite the fact that in this same group of patients, the authors failed to find any differences in plasma levels of FSH, LH, oestradiol and testosterone in women with psychosexual problems, compared with a matched group of women, without dyspareunia or loss of libido — a finding that concurs with that of Hallstrom (1977).

However, Dow et al. (1983), in a carefully designed and executed double blind controlled trial of this treatment package, failed to replicate Studd's findings. These authors, whose methodology is difficult to fault, found an equally significant improvement in all measures of sexual behaviour for both oestradiol implant alone and the combined oestradiol-testosterone implant. Table 4.4 illustrates these results in respect of three

Table 4.4

Pre and Posttreatment Scores for Three Measures of
Sexual Behaviour, Vasomotor and Psychological Symptoms

Measure	Treatment	Pre	Post (6 months)
Sexual Interest	O	2.4	3.8
	O + T	1.8	3.5
Sexual satisfaction	O	2.5	4.4
	O + T	2.3	5.1
Sexual responsiveness	O	2.0	3.6
	O + T	1.5	3.5
Vasomotor symptoms	O	7.8	4.0
	O + T	8.0	3.1
Psychological symptoms	O	26.2	18.1
	O + T	21.6	11.7

O = Oestradiol; T = Testosterone
Adapted from Dow et al. (1983)

of these measures. Concomitant with this improvement in sexual functioning, these authors also report, a marked improvement for both groups in all other climacteric symptomatology — vasomotor, somatic and psychological. These improvements led them to suggest that 'both treatments may have been equally effective in enhancing libido as an indirect function of the control of vasomotor symptoms and an increase in general wellbeing after oestradiol replacement' (p.365). Thus, under double blind conditions, the oestradiol alone was as effective as the combined implant, indicating that the efficacy of the latter in the reports by Studd and his colleagues may have been a placebo or a domino effect. Once again, it would appear that we have an example of the ubiquitous effect relief of vasomotor can have on all other complaints, including those of sexual dysfunction.

On the basis of the empirical evidence therefore, one can only but agree with the conclusion of van Keep and Gregory (1977) in their discussion of sexual relations in the ageing female in Money and Musaph's *Handbook of Sexology*:

> Folklore competes with findings on the immediate impact of the menopause on a woman's erotic interest and practice, but there is no evidence that the hormonal changes around the time of the menopause have any direct influence on a woman's libido. It is rare to have complaints of frigidity beginning all of a sudden with the menopause and, as at any age level, such sudden complaints are generally attached to a host of other complaints about family and marriage. If a woman does find her sexual interest waning in the post-menopausal period, the cause very likely lies in life-history factors or the influence of the fatigue, vaginal atrophy and other symptoms of the climacteric (p.843).

4.3. PSYCHIATRIC ILLNESS DURING THE CLIMACTERIC

Psychiatry is the specialist branch of medicine which deals with the diagnosis, treatment and management of mental and nervous disorders. Within clinical psychiatry there has developed a diagnostic system in which conditions are classified on the basis of the presenting symptoms, their natural history and, where possible, their aetiology. This system is now laid out in the *International Classification of Diseases* within the sections coded 290 to 319 (World Health Organisation, 1977).

In this section we shall examine the psychiatric literature for evidence of an association between the climacteric and menopause, and such formally diagnosable psychiatric disorders. By this is meant a recognised syndrome with its own natural history and clinical picture for which the climacteric has some aetiological significance. Conditions of this sort may not be detected in general population surveys of climacteric symptoms, partly because of their rarity and partly because the methods used in these surveys would not be appropriate. Furthermore, women with such conditions would tend to be referred to psychiatric agencies rather than gynaecology or menopause clinics. It is true that Ballinger (1975) reported a high level of psychiatric morbidity among climacteric women in the survey in Dundee. This, however, was of a minor variety and certain criticisms have been made of the method of identifying cases, and the confounding of psychiatric with climacteric symptoms (section 3.2). This point will be returned to at the end of this section. To examine the association of formal psychiatric illness and the climacteric we must turn to psychiatric sources.

Involutional Melancholia

Indeed, in clinical psychiatry there exists a long tradition associating formal psychiatric illness with the climacteric period. The condition, known as involutional melancholia, is described with precision in the early classical textbooks of psychiatry and is based on the idea that among women the menopause may have significant psychological and physiological effects that lead to serious clinical depression in predisposed individuals. Its early importance is reflected in the work of the eminent German psychiatric nosologist Kraepelin, in the fifth edition of whose textbook *Psychiatrie*, involutional psychoses formed, together with dementia praecox and manic depressive psychosis, one of the three major categories into which the functional psychoses were subdivided. Rosenthal (1968), in a historical review of the syndrome, describes the classical picture as follows:

> An involutional psychotic depression is a depressive episode of major proportion occurring for the first time in the involutional ages without a prior history of manic depressive illness .... The onset is gradual, with a slow buildup of hypochondriasis, pessimism, and irritability, finally flowering into a full-blown depressive syndrome. The most prominent features are motor agitation and restlessness, a pervading affect of anxiety and apprehension, an exaggerated hypochondriasis (sometimes with bizarre delusions), and occasional paranoid ideation which infrequently dominates. These distinguishing symptoms may be thought of as superimposed on a basic depressive substrate with insomnia, anorexia, and weight loss, and feelings of guilt and worthlessness. The depressed affect is described by some as shallow as compared to that seen in other depressive patients. Retardation is often described as absent or masked by the agitation' (p.23).

From the very beginning, however, the notion of a specific involutional entity, such as that described above, has been challenged, notably by Dreyfus (1907), who based his criticisms on an extensive follow up of the actual cases Kraepelin used to formulate the syndrome originally. Over the years since, major figures in psychiatry (Henderson and Gillespie, 1932; Lewis, 1934; Mayer-Gross et al., 1955) have contributed to the controversy as to whether involutional melancholia or depression exists as a distinct syndrome with its own aetiology, natural history and clinical picture. Gradually the balance of orthodox psychiatric opinion has become opposed to the notion of a distinct involutional condition, given expression in the statement by Martin Roth that 'the concept of a specific involutional pattern of endogenous depression .... is no longer tenable' (Roth, 1959, p.53).

Much of the controversy in early years was based on arguments derived from personal clinical experience and reports of series of cases. Some harder evidence opposed to the notion of a specific involutional depressive condition comes from a systematic study by Tait et al. (1957). These authors carried out a review of 54 first admission female patients within the age range 40 to 55 years to a Scottish psychiatric hospital. Symptoms, and what are described as background information, were recorded for all patients. It was firstly found that the latter (family history of mental illness, possible precipitating factors, age of menarche, marital status, sexual adjustment, past physical illness, personality characteristics etc) all failed to distinguish these patients from normal women of the same age. Nor, within the patient group, did they distinguish 29 women diagnosed as having a primary depression from those with psychoneuroses. Furthermore, the 29 depressed women did not seem markedly distinct, symptomatically, from depressed women of other ages, and it was with regard to the purely depressive aspects of their conditions only, that they differed from the neurotic patients in the group.

The authors therefore concluded that these depressed climacteric women were neither clinically of the classical involutional mould, nor were they aetiologically different from non-depressed patients presenting at the same biological period. They further concluded that 'any contribution of the involutional period to the clinical picture of depression may be accidental or at best pathoplastic and the origins of the depression itself, therefore, remains just as autonomous as that of other endogenous psychoses' and further that there were good reasons 'for believing the boundaries of this traditional syndrome are more nebulous than those of other diagnostic groups' (p.143).

Another source of empirical evidence regarding the possible existence of a typical involutional syndrome are factor analytic studies of depressive symptoms. This is a statistical technique based on correlational methods which allows the identification of clusters of symptoms, perhaps reflecting different types of depression (see section 7.4 for a fuller account of this technique). Numerous factor analytic studies of depressive symptomatology have been carried out over the years, for example by Hamilton (1960), Friedman et al. (1963), Kiloh and Garside (1963), Rosenthal and Klerman (1966), Rosenthal and Gudeman (1967), Kendell and Gourlay (1970), Roth et al. (1972) and Kiloh et al. (1972). None have produced a cluster of symptoms corresponding to those making up the classical involutional syndrome, these symptoms tending to be subsumed within the more orthodox syndromes of reactive and endogenous depression. Furthermore, Rosenthal and Gudeman (1967) could find no differences between psychiatrically depressed women, aged between 40 to 59 years and those between 25 to 39 years, in average scores on those symptoms supposedly making up the involutional syndrome. Nor could they differentiate these age groups on any other variables.

This and other evidence prompted Saul Rosenthal, the distinguished American psychiatrist, in an influential and comprehensive review of literature up to that time (Rosenthal, 1968) to note 'a definite paucity of involutional melancholia patients in current populations' and to doubt whether the syndrome really exists, or ever did exist, as a distinct clinical entity. Rosenthal writes:

> It is suspected that under the psychological and social stresses of the involutional years, depressive illness may emerge in many different kinds of patients and in varying degrees of severity. They might include patients with obsessive, hypochondriacal and hysterical life patterns and others with first or recurrent episodes of manic depressive illness' (p.33).

This statement implies that psychiatric breakdown during the climacteric may take various forms depending on the predisposing characteristics of the individual and may, in many cases, constitute the recurrence of a previous psychiatric disorder.

In the second edition of the official *Diagnostic and Statistical Manual of Mental Disorders* of the American Psychiatric Association (1968), involutional melancholia is characterised by three distinguishing criteria — the symptom picture, absence of a previous depressive episode and absence of precipitating life stress. These three criteria were examined by Weissman (1979) in a group of 422 consecutive female patients with a diagnosis of major non-polar depression who presented at the Yale University Depression Research Unit. These women were divided into three groups — premenopausal, younger than 45 years; menopausal, aged 45 to 55 years; and postmenopausal, 56 years or older.

The symptom patterns of patients in these three groups were firstly compared. There were no differences between the groups in sleep disturbance, anxiety, depression, apathy, somatisation, delusions or overall severity of depression. Women in the involutional period did not therefore show a distinct symptom pattern. These results were replicated by other clinical and patient self report measures used in the study. Nor were there any statistical differences between menopausal women and the other two groups in regard to a history of previous depressive episodes — the second criteria. In addition a global judgement was made by a psychiatrist in the first 157 cases as to whether family, social or other personal stress was present at the onset of the depression, and whether stress was a precipitatory factor in the depression. Again no significant differences emerged between the menopausal women and the other two groups.

Thus, none of the three criteria, distinguishing depression during the menopause from that occurring at other times, was fulfilled. Figures for two of the criteria are shown in Table 4.5 which indicates that these

Table 4.5

*Percentages of Depressed Women having two
of the DSMM Criteria for Involutional Depression*

Depression Occurring	Absence of Previous Episode	Absence of Life Stress
Before menopause	44	18
During menopause	47	26
After menopause	65	46

Adapted from Weissman (1979)

criteria are associated more with chronological age, than with the menopause. Once again characteristics thought to be associated with the menopause are shown to be part of the general ageing process (section 4.1). On the basis of this study Weissman concluded that there was 'no support for the validity of involutional melancholia as a distinct diagnostic entity' (p.744). It should be noted that involutional melancholia, as defined above, has been excluded from the third edition of the *Diagnostic and Statistical Manual of Mental Disorders*.

Other Psychiatric Disorders

Nevertheless, the belief has persisted among some psychiatrists (for example, Osofsky and Seidenberg, 1970) that even if there is no clinically distinct involutional syndrome, the risk of formal psychiatric illness, and in particular some form of depression, was greater during the climacteric than at other times of life. Recent evidence indicates that this belief is also without foundation.

Empirical evidence opposed to this viewpoint comes from a study by Winokur (1973). This author studied a group of women, all of whom had an affective disorder either before or after the menopause, to determine if there was a greater risk of depression during the menopause than at other times of the life span. The women consisted of 76 consecutive hospital admissions with a psychiatric diagnosis of affective disorder. Defining an affective episode occurring during the menopause as one in which there had been a hospitalisation within three years of the age the patient gave for the occurrence of the menopause, it was found that there was a 7.1 per cent risk of developing an affective disorder during the menopause, and a six per cent risk during all other times. This difference was not significant. Winokur concluded that 'from the current data the menopause does not seem to be an important factor in precipitating an episode of affective disorder. That it has been so considered may well be the result of the chance association of menopause and affective disorder and of a third factor, age' (p.93).

Winokur's study, although a careful one, was carried out on a fairly small sample of patients. However, over the years the findings of large scale epidemiological studies of psychiatric disorder, in which data relating to the climacteric years has been reported, tend to support his conclusions. For example, Hagnell (1966), in a ten year longitudinal study in Sweden, found no support for an increase in mental disorders, particularly neuroses during the climacteric. Adelstein et al. (1968) in a study of adult psychiatric patients derived from a case register in Salford, England, over a five year period, found no evidence from inception rates to support the notion of an increase in depression associated with the involutional period. Similar results have been reported from the longitudinal community survey carried out in New Haven in the United States (Weissman and Myers, 1978), in which no evidence was found of an increase in depressive symptoms in women around the menopausal years.

Perhaps the most definitive epidemiological study of psychiatric disorder at the climacteric is that conducted in Sweden by Hallstrom (1973, 1977). This study has already been referred to in the preceding section on sexual functioning during the climacteric. Between 1968 and

1970 more than 800 women between the ages 38 and 60 years were surveyed to determine possible changes in mental health during the climacteric. No significant differences were found in the incidence of mental illness, depressive illness nor psychiatric morbidity in general, in the different age strata, as a function of the menopause.

Like Rosenthal (1968) in regard to the existence of a specific involutional syndrome, Weissman and Klerman (1977), of the Depression Research Unit at Yale, in the course of a major review, this time of sex differences and the epidemiology of depression, arrived at a similar conclusion regarding depression in general, noting that there was 'no evidence that women are at greater risk from depression during the menopausal period or that depression occurring in this period has a distinct clinical pattern' (p.106).

Finally, many writers in the past have noted that women presenting at the climacteric with a diagnosable psychiatric illness tend to have a previous history of psychiatric problems (Stern and Prados, 1946; Donovan, 1951; Fessler, 1950). More specifically Greenhill (1946) found that in a group of women referred to a psychiatric clinic with the 'menopausal syndrome', of those who could be identified as having a definite psychiatric condition, for a quarter the symptoms were life long, and another quarter were suffering from a relapse of a psychiatric illness that had previously remitted.

The failure to find any association between the climacteric period and formal psychiatric illness does not exclude the possibility that during that time some women may experience an increase in symptoms of a *psychological* nature. This has been clearly demonstrated in Chapter 3, in the review of general population surveys of symptoms. What is being argued is that during the climacteric, few of these women experience these symptoms at a level of severity or of a quality, that would justify a psychiatric diagnosis or referral to a psychiatric agency. Nor, for that matter can these non-specific psychological symptoms be accounted for by an increase in psychiatric morbidity. A few women might however, experience symptoms at a level of severity that a psychiatrist might well describe as being at a case or a borderline case level. At a certain level of severity however, the dividing line between what is clinical and subclinical is a fine, and at times, arbitrary one.

This is one of the problems arising in the definition of cases in psychiatric epidemiology, previously referred to in section 3.2 when discussing the survey by Ballinger (1975) of psychiatric morbidity at the menopause. In using the General Hospital Questionnaire, Ballinger chose to label climacteric women who reported more than a certain number of symptoms as 'psychiatric cases'. The difficulty here is that a quantitative measure of symptoms only, is being used to arrive at a psychiatric diagnosis, which is normally a clinical judgement based not only on the number of symptoms but their nature, severity, history and the circumstances surrounding them. See Wing et al. (1978) and Williams et al. (1980) for a fuller discussion of the problems of case definition in psychiatric epidemiology.

Notwithstanding the possibility of a few women with climacteric symptoms being categorised as having minor psychiatric disorders at that time, it would appear that from the standpoint of orthodox clinical psychiatry, the climacteric in general and the menopause in particular are not associated with any specific psychiatric syndrome, nor do they *provoke* major psychiatric disorder in women without a previous history of psychiatric complaints.

4.4. SUMMARY AND CONCLUSION

The evidence regarding those changes which occur in other aspects of women's functioning during the climacteric in general, and at the menopause in particular, can now be summarised.

1. Adverse changes, when they do occur during the climacteric, tend to be confined to more personal physical and psychological functioning rather than to attitudes, interests and social relationships within a wider setting.
2. Furthermore these changes tend to occur in functions which are already declining rapidly with age, such as, for example, the IHF index of Subjective Adaptation. Certainly, in comparison with age related changes, the changes in women's functioning at the time of the menopause specifically are relatively benign.
3. A similar phenomenon is observed with regard to sexual interest and activity, where the evidence suggests that any such decline during the climacteric is largely age related. This decline in sexual behaviour may however be exacerbated at the menopause. When this does occur, it often represents the accentuation of pre-existing sexual inadequacy, the recurrence of an earlier difficulty, or is associated with other adverse social and interpersonal factors.
4. Studies of loss of libido following surgical menopause in younger women, where age is less likely to be a confounding factor, indicate that in these cases any loss or decline of sexual

interest or performance is likely to have psychological, rather than hormonal origins. When sexual dysfunction improves following oestrogen therapy this appears, as in the case of non-vasomotor complaints, either to be a placebo effect or be secondary to the relief of vasomotor symptoms.
5. As far as formal psychiatric illness is concerned the view that there exists a specific and distinct involutional syndrome is no longer tenable. The bulk of psychiatric opinion has swung firmly against the view that there is a form of psychiatric illness peculiar to the menopause or climacteric period of life.
6. Nor is there any evidence of an increase in other formal psychiatric disorders in association with the climacteric. When such disorders do occur during the climacteric they are coincidental, or there is often a previous history of psychiatric breakdown in women of vulnerable predisposition. Thus at the most the climacteric may serve to provoke the recurrence of a previous psychiatric condition.

Conclusion

Whilst there is consistent evidence that the time of the climacteric is associated with an elevation of non-specific physical and psychological symptoms, the evidence is less clear that adverse changes occur in other aspects of women's social and psychological functioning to any *widespread* degree. Those changes which do occur tend to be confined to immediate physical and psychological functioning, which to some extent could be seen merely as extensions of the symptomatic increase. Moreover, when such adverse changes do take place they tend to do so in functions which are already declining with age. This is especially so in the case of sexual behaviour, dysfunction of which is often further associated with a previous history of sexual inadequacy and other pre-existing social and psychological problems. In addition, the notion of a specific involutional psychiatric disorder peculiar to the climacteric period is no longer tenable, nor can climacteric symptoms be accounted for by an increase in psychiatric disorders in general. Again, when psychiatric illness does occur at that time, it often does so among women with a previous history of psychiatric problems.

Thus, during the climacteric the tendency is for any age related decline in social and psychological functioning to be *accelerated*, for already existing problems to be *accentuated* and for previous difficulties to *recur*. From an aetiological standpoint therefore, the climacteric in general, and the menopause in particular, do not function as primary aetiological factors but act in a more indirect exacerbating manner.

# 5

Psychosocial Determinants of Women's Responses During the Climacteric

Towards the end of Chapter 1, climacteric symptoms and complaints were considered, following the proposals of Utian and Serr (1976), to derive from three major sources — oestrogen deficiency, sociocultural factors and psychological factors. It has been established in Chapters 2 and 3 that the only symptoms which there are good reasons for believing have a hormonal basis and which show a close temporal relationship to the menopause are the symptoms of vasomotor instability and atrophic vaginitis. It has also been established in Chapters 3 and 4, that although the notion of a multi-symptom menopausal syndrome must be rejected, there is nevertheless good evidence that during the climacteric period in general there is an increase in a variety of non-specific physical and psychological symptoms, and that other adverse psychological changes may occur in women, to all of which may be applied the term 'climacteric syndrome'. In this and the following chapter we shall examine the research evidence regarding the part played by these 'sociocultural and psychological factors' in the origins of these symptoms and changes. We begin in this chapter by first considering those coincident psychosocial events which may be taking place during middle age and examine evidence of their association with symptom prevalence and other adverse reactions at that time. This will be followed by a review of the evidence regarding the effect pre-existing sociodemographic factors have on women's responses during the climacteric. Thus, having established in the two preceding chapters what psychological changes take place in women during the climacteric, we now begin the exercise of building an empirically based causal model, this being the second objective of this book (see Preface). In this chapter therefore, psychological and social factors are being regarded as independent variables and it is their effects on the dependent variables, described in the previous two chapters, which will be examined.

5.1. PSYCHOSOCIAL TRANSITION

A common theme in the literature is that the climacteric occurs just at a time in the life cycle when a variety of coincidental changes may be taking place in a woman's domestic, interpersonal and social situation. Writing on the social and psychological aspects of the 'Middle Years' in Arieti's *American Handbook of Psychiatry*, Neugarten and Datan (1974) list the major events that characterise the middle period of the life span as 'the launching of children from the home, the death of parents, climacterium, grandparenthood, illness, retirement and widowhood' (p.593). Regardless of the effect the climacteric may have, such events in themselves are usually seen as altering the woman's social role and status and as necessitating a degree of psychological and social readjustment. For some individuals, it is said, this may be a stressful experience as it may require them to undergo profound changes with respect to their perceptions of themselves, their current life situation and their future.

These views have their parallels in 'life cycle', 'life-course' or 'life-span' theories of change and development in adulthood (e.g. Neugarten, 1968; Vaillant, 1977; Levinson, 1978), which have earned the more fashionable label of 'mid-life crisis' in the popular literature (Sheehy, 1976; Gould, 1978). It is not the intention of the present writer to examine the validity or otherwise of these theories, recent interpretations of which, in relation to the middle aged women in general, are given in Neugarten (1979) and Rossi (1980). Their relevance in the present context is that they have given rise to an alternative or complementary view of the causation of the symptoms presented by women during the climacteric. This view is that many of these complaints are not due to hormonal and other biological changes and their consequences alone, but some may be attributed to difficulties in adjusting to the loss of old, and the demands or absence of new social roles (Bart and Grossman, 1978; Notman, 1979).

Others consider that should these events or role changes occur in conjunction with the menopause and its biological consequences, then the outcome may be all the more adverse. In addition, some of the role changes may in themselves be a direct result of the menopause, such as for example, the loss of reproductive function. This viewpoint is aptly expressed in the following quotation taken from Crawford and Hooper (1973), two of the leading proponents of this position:

> Whatever may be happening to a middle-aged woman's reproductive organs, biochemically and physiologically, equally important events in fact are taking place in the woman's socio-psychological situations and the menopause thus indeed signifies a *change* in her *life* of which the body changes are only a part. (p.469).

These authors conceptualise the coinciding of the biological changes and these sociopsychological events as a period of 'psychosocial transition', a term originally coined by the social psychiatrist Murray Parkes (Parkes, 1971) to refer to 'changes in the life space which take place over a relatively short period of time and which affects large areas of the assumptive world' (p.103). The changes in the life space which are usually highlighted in the case of the climacteric are those relating to the women's immediate family, marital relationships and domestic situation, most notable among which is the departure of children from home — the so-called 'empty nest syndrome'. Central to the notion of climacteric psychosocial transition therefore, is that the climacteric coincides with the occurrence of a number of changes in a woman's life situation and that it is these, rather than the internal biological changes, which are responsible for much climacteric distress. The question now arising is what empirical evidence exists to support these and other similar contentions?

5.2. STUDIES OF PSYCHOSOCIAL TRANSITION

The foregoing themes were touched upon in some of the surveys of symptomatology already discussed in Chapter 3. Ballinger (1975), for example found that 'psychiatric cases' among her sample of Dundonian women, had a fair amount of domestic and family problems. Psychiatric cases tended to have larger families, some 45 per cent having three or more children as against 30 per cent of non-cases. In response to a question about particular family problems occurring in the past year, 45 per cent of cases and only 23 per cent of non-cases reported such problems, these mainly having to do with children, husband and ageing parents, in that order. Departures of children from home were also higher among cases than non-cases but not strikingly so, the figures being 33 per cent and 24 per cent respectively. It is difficult, however, to escape the conclusion, even given some dubiety over the classification of women as psychiatric cases, that some of these problems may well have been longstanding ones in a vulnerable group of women.

Bungay et al. (1980) in their survey of symptoms in relation to age among Oxford women, also noted that more women in their forties and fifties reported events relating to children, such as leaving home, marrying or causing special worry, than did younger or older women. Furthermore, these events were positively associated with symptoms, an association which occurred throughout the climacteric age range. However, no details are given about the method of eliciting this information, nor is any data presented, so that it is not possible to gauge the magnitude of these effects on symptoms.

In both these surveys these themes had been dealt with in a somewhat perfunctory manner and secondary to the main objective of the survey which was to ascertain symptom prevalence at the time of the menopause. However, in two other symptom surveys, those by van Keep and Kellerhals (1974) and Holte and Mikkelsen (1982), more systematic examinations had been carried out of the effect such psychosocial factors might have on women during the climacteric. These, together with some other empirical studies specifically investigating these themes will now be reviewed in some detail. These studies are listed in Table 5.1 which summarises the method and outcome of each. The main aspect of psychosocial transition which has preoccupied investigators has been the effect the departure or absence of children from home have on climacteric women and this, in various ways, has been a feature of all studies. As can be seen, as in other areas of climacteric research, studies vary considerably

Table 5.1

Summary of Studies Investigating Effects of Psychosocial Factors on Climacteric Women

Authors	Location	Source of Sample	Size and Age	Menopausal Status	Outcome Measures	Factors Not Related to Outcome Measures	Factors Related to Outcome Measures
Van Keep and Kellerhals (1974)	Zurich, Switzerland	Random sample	448 46—55	Jaszmann's criteria	Climacteric index, other functions (see Table 4.1)		Absence of children during premenopause
Holte and Mikkelsen (1982)	Drammen, Norway	Community register	139 45—55	McKinlay's criteria	Six symptom factors	Absence of children from home	Quality of social network
Crawford and Hooper (1973)	Bristol, England	Church groups, press, clinics	106	Self defined	Self reported symptoms	Departure of children, arrival of grandchild, marital adjustment	
Lowenthal and Chiriboga (1979)	San Francisco, USA	Not reported	27 middle age	Not determined	Life evaluation chart	Pre-empty nest	
Krystal and Chiriboga (1979)	San Francisco, USA	Not reported	45 middle age	Not determined	Morale scale, activity checklist	Stages of child rearing	
Scheider and Brotherton (1979)	Melbourne, Australia	Menopause clinic	20 39—58	Clinical examination	Beck depression inventory	Loss of reproductive function, empty nest, ageing parents, deaths	Marital problems, economic difficulties, problems in adolescence, role impairment
Uphold and Susman (1981)	USA	Clubs, churches	185 40—60	Jaszmann's criteria	Symptom scale	Stages of child rearing	Marital adjustment

in methodology. The outcome methods are, however, for the most part the same as or similar to those employed in studies reviewed in the preceding two chapters.

Van Keep and Kellerhals (1974)

In the course of the IHF Swiss survey, information had been obtained as to whether women had children at home or not, designated as 'maternal role'. Total Climacteric Index scores of women within the 46-55 year age range, were reported according to maternal role for each of the three menopausal status groups. In the case of the peri and postmenopausal group there was little difference in symptom severity between women with or without children at home. However, a striking feature was that during the premenopause, those women without children at home had considerably higher symptom scores than those with children. In fact premenopausal women without children at home, had the most severe symptoms of all the subgroups, as can be seen in Figure 5.1. This, the authors refer to as an 'anticipated climacteric', thereby implying that the departure of children in the early climacteric, before the actual event of the menopause, may prematurely precipitate symptoms normally experienced later. This, as we shall see, is in fact the only study to demonstrate any association between the absence or departure of children from home and symptoms. It suggests that any negative response to the departure of children from home may have little to do with the menopause and may indeed be more distressing should it occur before that event.

The effect of maternal role on the various social and psychological characteristics listed in Table 4.1 was also examined in this study (IHF, 1975). Having no children at home exercised little influence on the great majority of these measures including Subjective Adaptation, the function which had been most adversely affected at the perimenopause. Where maternal role did exercise an effect, this was for fairly obvious and innocuous reasons, such as cultural activities and social contacts being curtailed among women with children at home. Women without children at home tended to evaluate the maternal role more highly and the presence of children reduced marital conflict. The former probably reflects a degree of nostalgia and the latter could be due to less opportunity for conflict, as a result of preoccupation with children. Maternal role, however, exercised these influences at all menopausal stages, although the effects tended to be accentuated at the perimenopause.

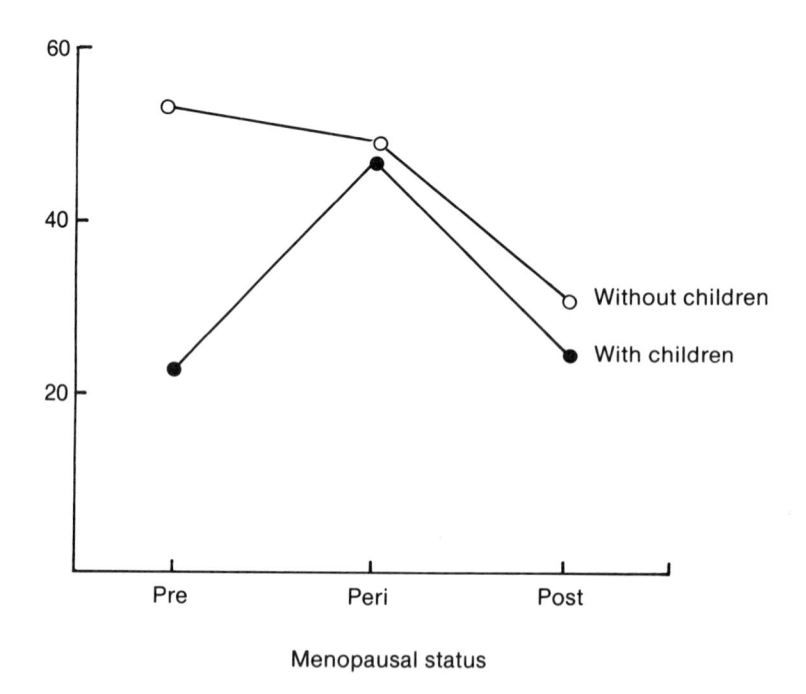

Figure 5.1 Percentage of women with climacteric index greater than eleven points in relation to menopausal status and maternal role.

(adapted from van Keep and Kellerhals, 1974)

Holte and Mikkelsen (1982)

The research team conducting the Norwegian Female Climacteric Project, the methodology of which has been previously described in section 3.2, also investigated the effect having children at home or not, had on their six factorially derived categories of symptoms. They also included a measure of the quality of a woman's current social network, as reflected in the number of friends and confiding relationships she had. While the symptom factors of mood lability and nervousness were high in women with limited social networks, *none* of the six categories of symptoms were associated with either the presence or absence of children at home. Thus, what were probably pre-existing social factors exercised an effect on symptoms, whereas psychosocial change, in the form of the departure of children from home, had no such effect.

Crawford and Hooper (1973)

We now turn to an earlier study by the two authors whose views on menopausal psychosocial transition have been described in section 5.1 of this chapter. In this study the authors set out specifically to test their hypothesis that 'there would exist complex relationships between the specific biological life event of the menopause and other psychosocial life events such as the two crises (as we have called them) in middle-age' (p.479). The two crises in question were the departure of a first child in marriage and the arrival of the first grandchild.

The data reported was based on a group of 43 women, living in the city of Bristol, whose first child or only child was about to marry, and 63 women who were expecting the arrival of their first grandchild. These women were contacted either through the local church, by studying the engagement columns of the local press, or through their daughters attending an ante-natal clinic. As might be expected this resulted in a sample highly biased towards the higher social classes. In addition the response rate of those initially contacted was for the postparental group only 15 per cent and for the grandparental group 42 per cent. The sample is therefore in no sense representative of the general population. Those co-operating were visited at home by an interviewer and asked a number of questions, about health, marital relationships and their feelings regarding the forthcoming wedding or birth. Menopausal status was determined by self evaluation. Those who regarded themselves as menopausal were asked to describe their symptoms and those who regarded themselves as postmenopausal to recall their symptoms when menopausal. Premenopausal women do not appear to have been asked about symptoms at all. In design this study is therefore an unusually poor one. Nevertheless, it is of interest to consider its main findings, which in general were negative.

The main interest of this study centred on the relationship between women's attitudes to the two 'psychosocial' events and menopausal status and symptoms. Attitudes of women to both events were rated as to whether these were positive, negative, neutral or anticipating no change. Women felt mostly negative or neutral (70 per cent) to the coming marriage, whereas in respect to the coming grandchild they were mostly positive or anticipated no change (82 per cent). In terms of the authors' hypothesis, that the menopausal experience would be 'intimately related to these role changes', it was expected that women who were experiencing the menopause would have more negative attitudes to both events and that women with such negative attitudes would have more symptoms.

In the event no association was found between any of the three variables — menopausal status, symptoms, or attitude to either event.

That is, women currently experiencing the menopause did not have a more negative attitude to these events, nor did women with a negative attitude to either event report more symptoms. Furthermore, although as many as 75 per cent of women felt that the forthcoming marriage was going to mean a change in their way of life, and 52 per cent felt similarly about the coming grandchild, neither menopausal status nor symptoms were related to these judgements in any way.

The only positive finding to emerge was that in the case of the forthcoming marriage symptoms were related to the sex of the offspring to be married. Here it was found that more women whose daughters were getting married reported symptoms than those whose sons were getting married, but this occurred regardless of menopausal status (see Table 5.2). However, neither birth order and age of the offspring being married,

Table 5.2

Number of Climacteric Women With and Without Symptoms in Relation to Sex of Marrying Child

	Without Symptoms	With Symptoms
Son	6	4
Daughter	2	14

Adapted from Crawford and Hooper (1973)

nor whether or not he or she was an only child were related to the presence and type of symptoms. Nor were there any association between the menopausal experience and other factors in the mother-child relationship, such as where the child was living before marriage, where he or she would be living afterwards, frequency of contact and the existence of other dependent children still living at home. Women had also been asked a number of questions relating to how they perceived their marital relations but again none of these features were associated in any way with menopausal status nor the reporting of symptoms.

The most striking finding emerging from this study therefore is the lack of any relationship between any of these variables (attitude to either psychosocial events, marital harmony, menopausal status) and symptoms. The authors' hypothesis has clearly not been substantiated since the evidence from this study, such as it is, is that being menopausal does not greatly influence women's feelings about and reaction to those events within the family which are regarded as 'crisis' points at this time of life. However, it must be borne in mind that this was a particularly poorly designed study.

Lowenthal and Chiriboga (1972)

In the next two studies to be considered in this section, the authors also set out to examine in some detail the impact of the departure of children from home (the 'empty nest' experience) on a group of both men and women in middle life. In this first study the subjects consisted of 27 men and 27 women of middle to lower middle class, approaching the 'empty nest' stage of parenthood; that is their youngest child was about to graduate from high school and leave home. Each subject was interviewed in depth in the course of which a number of questionnaires and rating scales were administered. The main measure consisted of a life evaluation chart by means of which the subjects rated different periods of their lives in regard to the satisfaction it had provided.

In the case of only three women was their present phase of life (the pre-empty nest phase) rated lowest relative to others, and in none of these cases did these low ratings have anything to do with the impending departure of their youngest child. Furthermore in response to direct questioning in interview, although for many, children and family continued to be a major source of satisfaction, extremely few saw the departure of children as a turning point in their lives or as a particular source of frustration. In those instances where such an event was described as a 'turning point', the child had departed from home under unhappy circumstances. While several women reported marital difficulties, none of them indicated that these problems were in any way connected with the impending empty nest situation. As far as sex differences were concerned, the responses of men were not dissimilar from women, except that as a group, men's mood and morale were more positive. This the authors attributed to 'a sex difference in affective proclivities'.

These authors conclude that 'neither responses to specific questions about critical periods and problems, nor the content of these detailed protocols as a whole convey the impression that the prospects of the departure of the youngest child are in any way threatening for this pre-empty nest sample' (p.14).

Krystal and Chiriboga (1979)

In a later study one of these authors (Chiriboga) carried out a further examination of the impact of the empty nest situation on men and women in middle life. This is an important and unique study because it is the only longitudinal study of its kind in this area. That is the subjects, 45 middle aged men and women, most of whom were expected to be exposed to the empty nest process, were followed up over a five year period as they went through this experience. Each subject was assessed initially, and again after 1½ and 5 years, using the 18 item Bradburn Morale Scale which is similar in content to symptom checklists used in other studies, and a 33 item Activity Checklist, designed by one of the authors. At each assessment point, which of three 'empty nest' conditions prevailing was determined for each subject. These were Full (all children still at home), Partial (at least one child had left home but not all) and Empty (all children left home).

The only significant difference to emerge for those experiencing a changing situation were as follows. Women changing from a Full to Empty nest situation showed a significant *decrease* in one of the 18 Morale Scales, namely depression, and women who had moved from a Partial to Empty situation also showed a similar decrease in depression and also in 'happiness'. For men the only significant change was that those in the Partial-Empty category became more 'excited'. There was no changes in activity level as situations changed. However, there was some evidence that activity level, when it did increase, did so during the Partial empty nest phase, and this occurred for both men and women. This is not surprising as the checklist dealt mainly with social and cultural activities.

These changes were interpreted by the authors as reflecting 'a readjustment within a transitory temporal process'. That is, those groups experiencing the early stages of the transition process (Full and Full-Partial groups) showed no significant changes in either activity level or morale. The Partial group, those slightly further into the process did show some changes. Groups fully into or through the process (Empty and Empty-Partial) however, showed greater changes in the form of increased activity and greater morale. This pattern of change suggests that women who are well into the transition, or who are fully through it, have reorganised their life styles to accommodate the increase in free time and change of role. None of this supports a 'crises theory' and the authors conclude that 'the overall impression obtained was one of positive rather than negative reactions to the empty nest and that the so-called crisis of the empty nest is more a collective myth than an experiential reality' (p.219).

Schneider and Brotherton (1979)

In this study of climacteric Australian women, a number of different psychosocial factors, including the departure of children from home, were examined in relation to women's responses at the menopause. The outcome measure, however, was not climacteric symptoms but the presence of psychiatric depression. The authors' aim was to determine those characteristics and circumstances which differentiated menopaual women who were depressed from those who were not. Their purpose was 'to gain an increased understanding of the ways in which certain physiological, social and psychological stresses may combine to contribute to the marked psychological morbidity in this particular phase (the menopause) of the female life cycle' (p.154). This not only seems to beg the question but also given the limitations of the study is somewhat ambitious in scope.

The group of women studied were selected from the first admissions to a menopause clinic of a Melbourne Hospital over a three month period. Women attending this clinic were either self referred or referred from an outside practice, and all presented with a variety of so-called typical menopausal symptomatology — tiredness, irritability, difficulty in making decisions, etc. They are therefore very much a clinical sample. The group studied consisted of 20 women within the age range 39 to 58 years, all married and all in good physical health. All were considered to be menopausal on the basis of their symptoms, gynaecological examination and relevant blood analyses. There is no indication that the now conventional time since last menstrual period was used in determining menopausal status. This group of women was in turn divided as to whether they were depressed or not on the basis of scores on the Beck Depression Inventory (Beck et al., 1961). These two sub-groups were then compared in regard to eight 'areas of stress', which had been elicited in the course of what seems to have been a semi structured interview designed 'to reveal information concerning a number of likely stresses discussed in the literature pertaining to psychological changes during the menopause' (p.154).

It was found that depressed women differed from those who were not in four of these areas of stress. Depressed women showed a significantly greater frequency of marital dissatisfaction, economic difficulty, early developmental disturbance and 'role impairment'. The last referred to a lack of interest or inability to function adequately either at work or in respect to interpersonal roles. Stress associated with the loss of the reproductive function, the care of aged parents, changes in parental role and precipitating factors, such as death or illness of loved ones, was not significantly different for the depressed and non-depressed groups. The authors conclude that their results support the view 'that premorbid functioning and personality are important predictors of a woman's ability to cope with the stresses of the menopausal period' (p.157). While one may possibly agree with the first part of this statement regarding the importance of premorbid functioning, the second part is less acceptable for the following reasons.

Firstly, these authors have not shown that the depression exhibited by these women had anything to do with their being menopausal, as no non-menopausal group was included of a similar age range. The sample is a highly selected clinical one, in which one would expect some degree of psychiatric morbidity (see introduction to Chapter 3). Furthermore, for reasons outlined in section 4.3, the current psychiatric view is that the time of the menopause or climacteric is not particularly associated with clinical depression nor, for that matter, with any other psychiatric condition. Secondly, they have shown that the depression exhibited by these women was not associated with any of those psychosocial factors thought to be peculiar to the climacteric period, such as loss of the reproductive function or loss of parental role. Nor was it associated with having to care for ageing parents or the death of loved ones. Thirdly, what they have shown is that psychiatric depression occurring at the climacteric among a clinical population of women was associated with more general pre-existing difficulties, such as marital and economic problems and problems during early development. Such factors are now known to be associated with depression in women at any age. See section 8.3 for a fuller discussion of the role of these factors in depression.

In brief, the significance of this study is that the authors have shown that depressive reaction, when it occurs at the time of the menopause, is not precipitated by psychosocial factors thought to be peculiar to that time, but is related more to general, chronic and *pre*-existing problems.

Uphold and Susman (1981)

As in the study by Krystal and Chiriboga (1979), these researchers also investigated the relationship between severity of symptoms in a group of climacteric women and *stages* of child rearing and in addition obtained a measure of marital adjustment. Although from the general population, the subjects were not a random sample but consisted of a group of 185 white middle class women all married, between the ages of 40 and 60 years. These women were contacted through civic and women's clubs and church organisations in six suburban communities in the Eastern United States.

The outcome measure was the 28 item checklist used by Neugarten and Kraines (1965) in their survey. In addition to total number of symptoms, a measure of total severity was obtained, using a four point scale to rate the reported severity of each symptom. Both these symptoms measures, therefore, combine vasomotor and non-vasomotor complaints. Child rearing stage was based on the presence or absence of children at home, there being three categories; the Prelaunching Stage, defined as the period when all children are at home; the Transitional Stage, covering the period between the time at least one child is gone and no children have been in the home for a period of one year, and the Empty Nest Stage, when no children have been at home for more than one year. Marital adjustment was measured by means of the Dyadic Adjustment Scale, a self administered rating scale which is both a reliable and valid measure of marital adjustment and is well documented (Spanier, 1976). Menopausal status was defined in terms of the criteria used by Jaszmann et al. (1969b). The design of this study is therefore a relatively good one.

The main positive finding was that for the group as a whole women low on marital adjustment had more numerous and more severe symptoms than those who had good marital relations. There was no evidence that child rearing stages were related to symptoms in any way. Women low on marital adjustment showed the same high frequency and severity of symptoms at all child rearing stages. These effects are illustrated for mean number of symptoms in Table 5.3 and appear quite convincing.

Table 5.3

Mean Number of Symptoms in Relation to Marital Adjustment and Child Rearing Stages

Child Rearing Stage	Marital Adjustment		
	Low	High	Total
Prelaunching	12.1	9.2	10.6
Transitional	13.3	10.1	11.8
Empty nest	12.5	10.0	11.2
Total	12.9	9.9	

Adapted from Uphold and Susman (1981)

So far these findings refer to the sample of women as a whole. Data was also reported for the group sub-divided according to menopausal status. Women low on marital adjustment had more numerous and more severe symptoms at all menopausal stages, and women who were menopausal had higher scores than those who were not. These effects can be seen in Table 5.4. As can also be seen, perimenopausal women of low marital adjustment had considerably more symptoms than might be expected. As the checklist included vasomotor ones, most of the increase

Table 5.4

Mean Number of Symptoms in Relation to Menopausal Status and Marital Adjustment

Menopausal Status	Marital Adjustment		
	Low	High	Total
Pre	12.7	9.6	11.2
Peri	21.5	12.7	17.1
Post	11.6	8.5	10.0
Total	12.6	9.6	

Adapted from Uphold and Susman (1981)

of symptoms in menopausal women is likely to be due to the known increase of such symptoms at that time (Chapter 3). This seems unlikely, however, to account for the extremely large rise in symptom frequency among perimenopausal women of low marital adjustment. The possibility exists, therefore, that the *exacerbation* of psychological symptoms which occurs at the menopause (Chapter 3) is considerably greater among women with poor marital relations, particularly in view of the fact that the authors state that there was no worsening of marital relations among women during the perimenopause.

The authors conclude that the quality of a woman's marriage is a potent factor in influencing her reactions during the climacteric, rightly pointing out that such a conclusion regarding marital relations per se must be tentative as poor husband and wife relations may be a reflection of poor emotional adaptation in general. Furthermore, it would appear that this influence may be particularly marked at the perimenopause, suggesting that at that time women experiencing poor marital relations are particularly vulnerable. Such factors may therefore contribute to the exacerbation which occurs at the perimenopause, not only of symptoms, but also of those other adverse reactions discussed in the preceding chapter. (See conclusion, section 4.4). Of added interest in this study is, of course, the failure once again to find any association between symptoms and the departure of children from home.

A summary of the outcome of the studies reviewed in this section can be found in Table 5.1, the most striking feature of which is the absence of any association between loss of parental role and negative reactions during the climacteric. What then is the basis of this widespread belief that there is such an association?

We have seen from the study by Lowenthal and Chiriboga (1972) that the departure of a child from home may in a few instances provoke a negative reaction, but only if the child has departed under unhappy circumstances. Others have also noted that negative reactions in response to children leaving home may be associated with the nature of relationships within the family. Levit (1963), in an unpublished doctoral thesis, reported that among a group of climacteric women, half of whom were past and half of whom were at the menopause, women who were high on 'motherliness' experienced greater anxiety at the menopause than similar women who were postmenopausal. Whether or not children were actually living at home made little difference to the level of anxiety. Levit concluded therefore, that the transition from childbearing to non-childbearing seemed to be more stressful to women who were highly invested in the motherly role than those who were not so invested in this role. Not dissimilar findings were reported by Bart (1971) among a group of depressed hospitalised climacteric women. Although this is clearly a highly selected and unrepresentative group of women, of some interest is the finding that the highest rate of depressive illness occurred among women experiencing maternal role loss who had overprotective or overinvolved relationships with their children. Clearly, on the occasions when the departure of children from home is associated with negative reaction during the climacteric, then this occurs in the context of highly unusual family relationships, which at times may aptly be described as pathological and are probably of relatively rare occurrence. It is these rare and more extreme cases, perhaps usually occurring among clinical populations, which have given rise to the widespread notion that loss of maternal role may precipitate adverse reactions in a substantial number of climacteric women.

5.3. SOCIODEMOGRAPHIC FACTORS

It is now well established on the basis of epidemiological studies, that broadly based demographic factors such as sex, social class, income level, employment status and educational attainment are associated with many physical, psychological and psychiatric conditions (see for example, Freeman et al., 1972; Morris, 1975; Tucket, 1976). This being so, the question arises as to what extent such factors may prove to be associated with the reactions of women during the climacteric. It has long been fashionable to regard preoccupation with the menopause as a phenomenon peculiar to the middle and upper classes of society. Yet, as we have seen in the section on sexual functioning (section 4.2) there was good evidence from the studies by Hallstrom (1973) in Sweden, van Keep and Kellerhals (1975) in Switzerland and Garde and Lunde (1981a,b) in Denmark that sexual difficulties at the climacteric were more common among women of lower socioeconomic status. In this section we shall examine the empirical research for evidence of an association between this, and similar factors, and symptoms reported by women during the climacteric. We shall begin by again returning to those surveys of symptom prevalence first discussed in Chapter 3, in some of which the influence of sociodemographic factors on symptoms was also investigated. In these surveys the commonest factors investigated have been social class, educational level, marital and employment status.

McKinlay and Jefferys (1974)

In this British survey these four sociodemographic factors, together with two other measures, number of live-born children (parity) and domestic workload, were examined in relation to symptoms by means of the method of cluster analysis used to examine relationships among symptoms. Graphical representation, similar to that shown in Figure 3.3, revealed that the points representing these six variables formed 'a loose cluster, at considerable distance from the remaining points' (p.109). This implies that in this sample of women, none of these characteristics was closely associated with either menopausal status or any of the symptoms. Furthermore, various cross-tabulations of these factors subsequently confirmed this general lack of association. At the outset, therefore, it looks as if these types of social factors have no influence whatsoever on climacteric symptomatology. However, in this respect the negative findings of this British survey differ from all others.

Jaszmann, Van Lith and Zatt (1969b)

The above researchers also examined symptoms in relation to four sociodemographic variables, these being income level, educational attainment, marital status and parity, in their survey of Dutch women. They found the overall number of complaints to be significantly higher in women of lower income, in women of lower educational level and in women who were married. These associations are shown in Table 5.5, and

Table 5.5

*Median Total Symptom Scores
in Relation to Sociodemographic Variables*

Variable		Pre	Peri	Post
Educational level	Low	3.1	4.3	3.1
	High	2.6	3.7	2.7
Income	Low	3.0	4.2	3.2
	High	2.7	3.9	2.7
Married	Yes	2.9	4.1	3.1
	No	1.8	3.7	2.5

(Menopausal Status columns: Pre, Peri, Post)

Adapted from Jaszmann et al. (1969b)

as can be seen exercise their effect within *all* menopausal status groups. As in the two UK surveys, number of pregnancies was unrelated to symptom frequency, although women who had never had children reported fewer symptoms. This last relationship, however, is obviously confounded by marital status. Clearly, then, the UK and Dutch studies are divergent in regard to the influence these three major sociodemographic factors of social class/income, educational level and marital status have on symptoms at the climacteric. The fourth factor, employment status, was not considered in the Dutch study.

The explanation for these discrepant findings between the British and Dutch surveys could be a statistical one however. Where differences in relation to socioeconomic variables were found in Jaszmann's study, they were, as can be seen from Table 5.5, of a fairly small magnitude. For example, menopausal women of low income reported a median of 4.2

complaints as opposed to 3.9 for women in the higher income bracket. This small difference is statistically significant presumably because of the very large numbers in each group — 536 and 459 respectively. In the UK studies such differences would have been unlikely to have attained significance because of the much smaller sizes of the groups. Thus the influence of sociodemographic variables on total symptoms counts in the Dutch study seems to be of a fairly small magnitude despite their statistical significance.

However, as no data is presented in this survey for vasomotor and non-vasomotor symptoms separately, differential effects of sociodemographic factors on different types of symptoms cannot be ascertained. In later studies of the effects of sociodemographic factors on symptoms, such distinctions have been made, with revealing results.

Greene and Cooke (1980)

One of these studies is the survey of Scottish climacteric women, which was also discussed in section 3.2. In that survey it will be recalled that non-specific somatic and psychological symptoms had been examined in relation to menopausal and climacteric status separately from vasomotor symptoms, using two symptom scales, derived from a factor analysis. Information had also been gathered at time of interview to allow subjects to be categorised according to socioeconomic status using the British Registrar General's classificatory system. No relationship was found between vasomotor symptoms and social class status but there was a marked association between the latter and other symptoms. This effect is illustrated in Figure 5.2 across climacteric status groups for both the somatic and psychological symptoms scales. This figure has been drawn on the basis of as yet unpublished data from that survey. There it can be seen that for both scales, mean symptom scores of women of low socioeconomic status increased moreso than those of women of high socioeconomic status during the climacteric and remained higher into the postclimacteric period. This effect is, however, greater for psychological symptoms, for which the class differences, during the late and postclimacteric, achieve statistical significance. These results, therefore, while being consistent with those of Jaszmann et al. (1969b), must cause one to reconsider the small magnitude of the association found by those authors between symptoms and social class and income level, as their symptom measures included vasomotor ones.

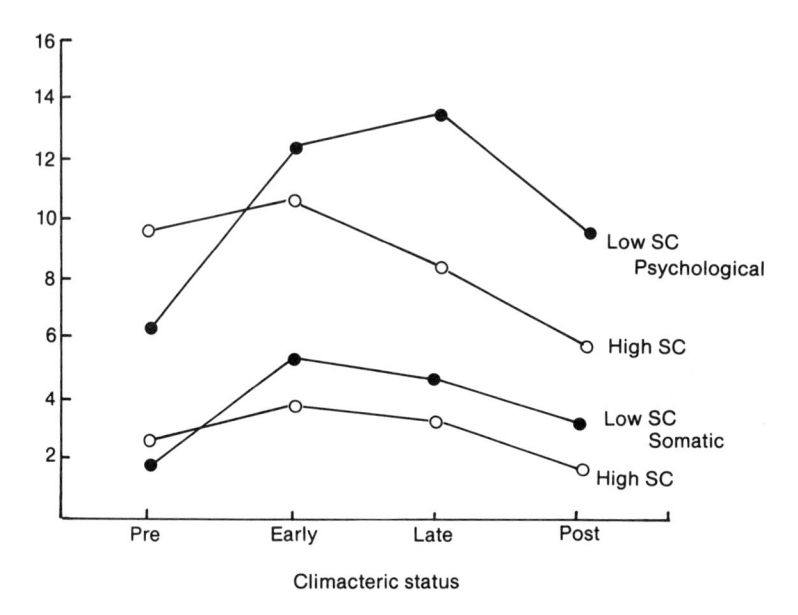

Figure 5.2 Mean scores on two symptom scales in relation to social class (SC).
(Greene and Cooke, 1980)

Campagnoli, Morra, Belforte, Belforte and Tousijn (1981)

A similar differential effect of socioeconomic status on symptoms was reported by the above authors in a study of Italian women. The study population consisted of 618 women, all of whom had undergone a natural menopause, living in the city of Turin. Data were collected by means of a postal questionnaire, the response rate being 56 per cent. In addition to information being available about their physical and socioeconomic status, these women were also asked about any symptoms they had experienced at the time of the menopause. These were divided into 'somatic' (hot flushes and sweating) and 'psychic' symptoms (anxiety, feeling depressed, irritability, crying spells), each being rated according to degree of severity. The results of this study are summarised in Table 5.6, which demonstrates that socioeconomic status had no effect on vasomotor symptoms, but that women of low status tended to report more severe psychological symptoms, than women of high status. These findings are, therefore, similar to those obtained by Greene and Cooke (1980).

Table 5.6

Percentage Incidence of Psychic and Somatic Symptoms in Relation to Socioeconomic Status

Socioeconomic Status	Somatic Symptoms			Psychic Symptoms		
	None	Slight Moderate	Severe	None	Slight Moderate	Severe
Low	18	62	20	22	56	22
High	18	64	18	30	56	14

Adapted from Campagnoli et al. (1981)

An interesting finding from this Italian study was that body weight was also differentially associated with types of symptoms in that light women had more somatic and heavy women more psychological symptoms. However, as the tendency for heavy women to have psychic symptoms was less marked in the lower socioeconomic group, the authors suggest that even here sociocultural factors, related to how the different classes evaluate weight, mediate to complicate the relationship between weight and symptoms. It is also generally considered that obesity and overeating frequently have a psychological basis. It should be noted that Jaszmann et al. (1969b) in their survey of climacteric symptomatology found no association between body type and total symptom count. This study by Campagnoli et al. (1981) therefore lends further force to the case for distinguishing between different types of symptoms and treating them separately.

Prill (1966)

In an earlier study of German women Prill (1966) had also obtained results contrary to those of Thompson et al. (1973) and McKinlay and Jefferys (1974), regarding the effect on climacteric symptoms of employment status, a factor not considered in the three preceding studies. Among German women it was found that of those with a part time job, only 8 per cent suffered from 'severe climacteric symptoms' compared with 24 per cent having no outside occupation. An important element in this relationship was the reason for working or not working. Prill (1977) observes that among women who had to work because of financial or other unwelcome reasons, and among those who wanted to work but because of circumstances, were not able to do so, symptoms were the most severe. As we shall see in later studies, simply lack of employment per se is probably not the main critical factor influencing symptoms.

Polit and Larocco (1980)

This was demonstrated in a much later study by Polit and Larocco (1980), the sole objective of which was the investigation of the association between frequency of symptoms during the climacteric and a variety of factors, including sociodemographic ones. As the title of the paper indicates it is a straight correlational study between symptom severity and possible aetiological factors in a sample of menopausal and postmenopausal women in the general population. This has the advantage that relationships are presented in terms of correlation coefficients which allows the magnitude of the effects to be seen. No data, however, is presented regarding the prevalence of symptoms in women of different menopausal status, but different types of symptoms were examined separately.

The group studied consisted of a sample of women between the ages of 40-60 years residing in an urban community in the Greater Boston area. The sample was randomly chosen using systematic sampling procedures and the data obtained by means of a postal questionnaire. Unfortunately, the return rate was only 33 per cent which is unusually low for this sort of exercise. This, therefore, throws some doubt on the representative nature of the informants. Furthermore, menopausal status was assigned using the unsatisfactory method of self determination, and the analysis of the data was based on the responses of 51 menopausal and 84 postmenopausal women combined. Symptoms were assessed by means of a short checklist of ten symptoms 'commonly associated with the menopause'. These included vasomotor symptoms, which were reported by 71 per cent of the women, as well as other physical and psychological symptoms. These symptoms were then examined in relation to educational level, employment status, marital status, religion, number of children, age of youngest child and family income.

Of these, only educational level and employment status showed any significant association with symptoms, women with a high level of educational attainment and women who were employed outside the home reporting fewer symptoms, thereby confirming the findings of Jaszmann et al. (1969b) and Prill (1966), respectively. The correlation between the total number of symptoms and educational level was 0.22 and that between employment status 0.25. Although these overall relationships are fairly modest, inspection of individual symptoms revealed that where sociodemographic variables were associated with symptoms, these were mainly psychological in nature, and that their effects on such symptoms could be fairly substantial. Table 5.7 illustrates the effect educational attainment had on two such symptoms. Vasomotor symptoms on the

Table 5.7
Percentage of Women Reporting Symptoms in Relation to Educational Attainment

Sympton	College Graduates	Non-College Graduates
Depression	19	64
Lack of energy	24	63
Vasomotor	No differences	

Adapted from Polit and Larocco (1980)

other hand showed no association with educational level. These differential effects on symptoms are similar to those obtained by Greene and Cooke (1980) and Campagnoli et al. (1981).

With respect to employment, part time workers tended to resemble non-employed women more than they resembled full time employees in their reporting of symptoms. In general, women working full time were less likely to report symptoms than women in the other two categories. For example, only 18 per cent of women working full time compared with 52 per cent of part time workers, and 45 per cent of non-employed women reported having trouble sleeping. Similar results were obtained with respect to other psychological symptoms. This confirms Prill's earlier observation that being employed per se is not the critical factor. What may be more important is that a woman is pursuing a full time career, rather than working on a part time basis with the object perhaps of supplementing the family income. Full time employment would obviously be facilitated by a higher level of educational attainment. Furthermore, it is probable that women of low social class who had a job outwith the home would not be pursuing a full time career and would not therefore experience the beneficial effect of career orientated employment.

Thus, this group of adverse sociodemographic factors — low social class, low educational level, low income and lack of full time employment

— could very well be interdependent and operate in unison. This would be consistent with the findings of an unpublished thesis by Lennon (1980), who noted that data from the U.S Health and Nutrition Examination Survey showed that 'women who occupy disadvantaged social positions, — specifically those with little education, the poor, the divorced and separated, and black women — are most likely to exhibit psychological distress whatever their menopausal status' (p.4182).

Holte and Mikkelsen (1982)

In the pilot study of the Norwegian Female Climacteric Project, previously discussed in sections 3.2 and 5.2, the six categories of symptoms used by those authors were also examined in relation to a number of sociodemograhic variables. These included educational level, financial and marital status and being employed. However, in this particular study the association between these factors and symptom categories were generally negative or of a modest level. The only positive relationships were that women whose husbands' income was low and who were not employed outwith the home tended to report more diffuse somatic symptoms. Thus once again income level and non-employment were found to be associated with non-specific symptoms, but in this instance only tenuously.

The authors account for these generally negative findings by suggesting that as Scandinavian countries are highly developed welfare states, relative to other Western industrialised societies, their populations are economically and culturally homogeneous at a generally high level of income. This is an interesting point because it follows that in those societies with a high standard of living, the effects of the climacteric may be relatively benign, and that where variation in response does occur, more sensitive social and psychological factors may be aetiologically more important. Indeed, in this particular study it was found that measures of previous 'menstrual coping' (pain, nausea, depression at menstruation) and the quality of a women's social network (see section 5.2) were more powerful predictors of psychological and general somatic symptoms than were sociodemographic factors.

Van Keep and Kellerhals (1974, 1975)

More detailed evidence of the effect that social class, and also employment, may have on a woman's reaction during the climacteric comes from the IHF surveys, already referred to in Chapters 3 and 4. In the Swiss study women were sub-divided into two social class groups on the basis of their husband's occupation. With the exception of the perimenopausal group, women of lower social class within all other four (age and menopause) groups had marginally higher Climacteric Index scores than those of higher social class, thereby indicating a fairly consistent but not large social class effect. However, as noted before, no separate analysis is provided in this index of vasomotor and non-vasomotor symptoms, and as we have seen from the studies by Polit and Larocco (1980), Greene and Cooke (1980) and Campagnoli et al. (1981), social class seems to influence psychological symptoms only.

That this may also be the case in the IHF Swiss study is demonstrated by the clear association between social class and the various other social and psychological characteristics listed in Table 4.1. Social class had a profound and widespread effect on almost all these measures. Women of lower social class consistently showed poor Subjective Adaptation at all ages and within all menopausal groups, this being particularly marked at the perimenopause. With regards to Role Identity, at almost all ages and

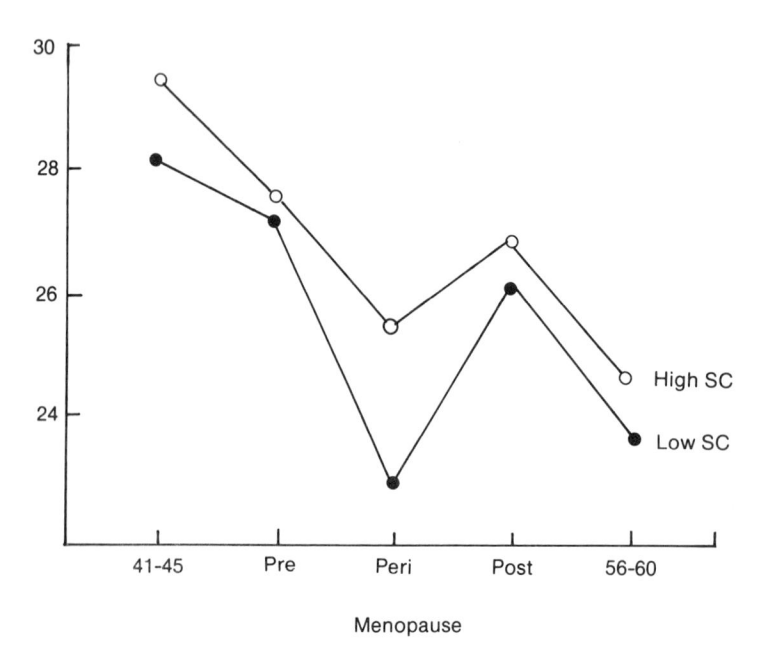

Figure 5.3 Index of subjective adaptation in relation to social class (SC) (adapted from van Keep and Kellerhals, 1974)

within all menopausal groups, women of lower social class evaluated all three traditional female roles (dependency, maternal and sexual) more highly than did women of higher social class. In the area of Immediate Family Relations women of lower social class tended to have a less satisfactory sex life, especially in the older age range, and marital and family disharmony tended to be greater among lower class women at all chronological and biological stages. It will be recalled that Hallstrom (1977) and Garde and Lunde (1980a,b) found a similar effect for social class on sexual functioning during the climacteric (section 4.2). Finally, all aspects of Wider Social Relations — cultural activities, social contacts and normative integration — were reduced in women of lower social class, again at all menopausal stages. Figure 5.3 serves to illustrate these effects in regard to Subjective Adaptation, which it will be recalled markedly declined during the climacteric, and Figure 5.4 in regard to

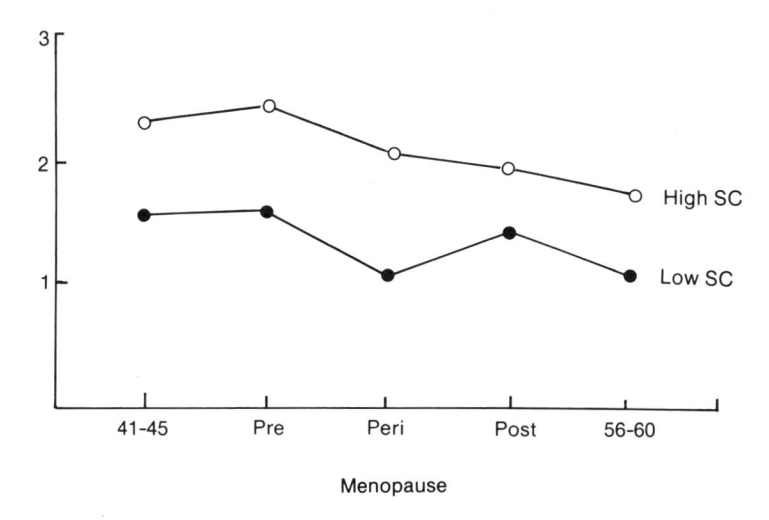

Figure 5.4 Index of cultural activities in relation to social class (SC) (adapted from van Keep and Kellerhals, 1975)

cultural activities, which changed little at that time. Comparing Figure 5.3 with Figure 4.1, it is clear that the dip in Subjective Adaptation at the perimenopause among climacteric women in general, was due largely to its greater decline in women of lower social class.

In summary, being of lower social class adversely affected almost all characteristics at all ages and throughout the climacteric. In addition the acceleration at the menopause in the decline of those functions already declining with age (section 4.1) is greater in women of low socioeconomic status. Some of these differences in social class, particularly those relating to role identity and wider social and cultural activities, probably reflect the more traditional concept women of lower class have of the female role. Nevertheless, of the four independent factors examined in the IHF Swiss study — age, menopausal status, maternal role and social class — the last named had the most profound and widespread adverse effect on climacteric women.

In the IHF Belgian survey it will be recalled that vasomotor and some other somatic symptoms (Circulatory Index) and psychological symptoms (Nervosity Index) were examined separately. It will also be

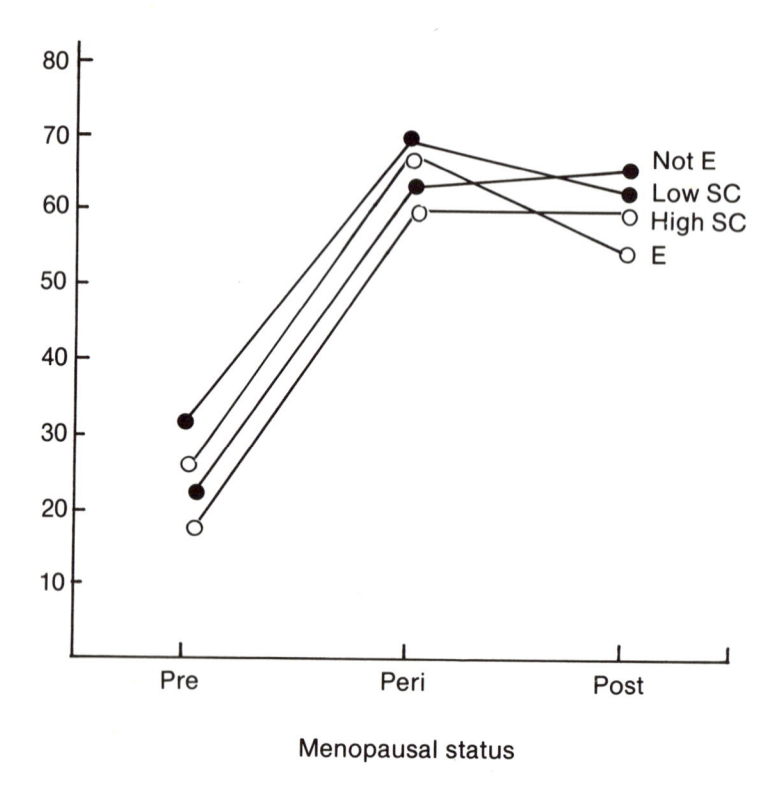

Figure 5.5 Percentage of women reporting flushes in relation to employment (E) and social class (SC).
(from Severne, 1979)

recalled that the former showed a considerably greater increase at the perimenopause than did the latter (see Figure 3.5). These symptoms were also examined separately in relation to social class and a second sociodemographic variable, employment status, defined as having a paid job outwith the home. It was found that vasomotor symptoms behaved quite differently from nervous ones in relation to these two sociodemographic factors. Vasomotor symptoms were essentially unrelated to either of these variables. This is illustrated for hot flushes in Figure 5.5 where it can be seen that little differences emerge between employed and non-employed women, or between women of different social class at any menopausal stage. All follow the same general pattern depicted earlier in Figure 3.5.

Quite a different picture emerged however in the case of nervous symptoms. These symptoms were related to both social class and

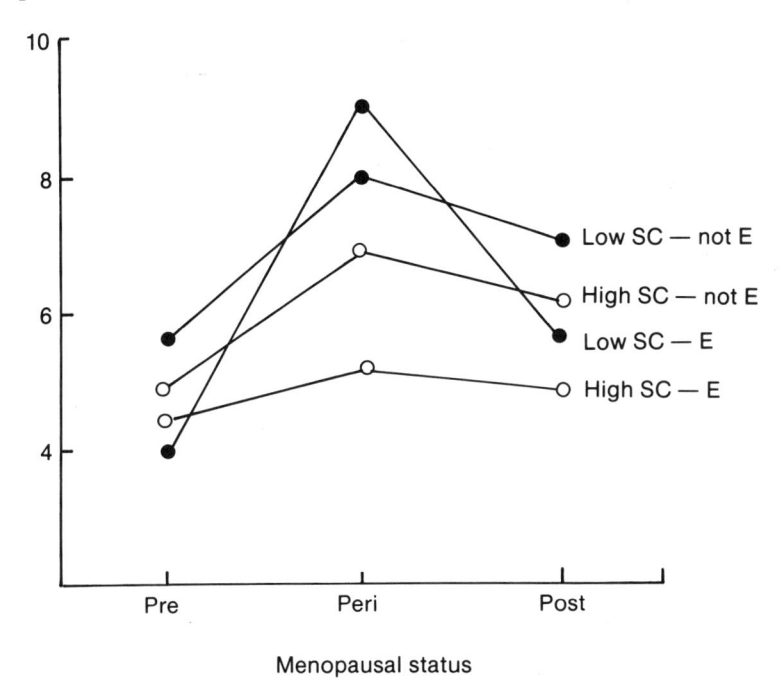

Figure 5.6 Mean scores on the nervosity index in relation to employment (E) and social class (SC)
(adapted from Severne, 1979)

employment status, but in a complex way, in that the effect of being employed depended on the social class of the women. This is illustrated in Figure 5.6 where the scores on the Nervosity Index of the four subgroups of women is seen at each menopausal stage to be quite disparate. It is clear from this figure that once again women of lower socioeconomic status had the more severe psychological symptoms at the time of the menopause. However among these women, those who were employed, experienced the more marked increase in symptoms at that time. In contrast among women of higher social class those employed had the least severe symptoms. In other words the effect of employment on symptoms is reversed depending on the socioeconomic status of the women. Thus the relatively smaller increase in psychological symptoms during the perimenopause among women in general (Figure 3.5) is shown to be due,

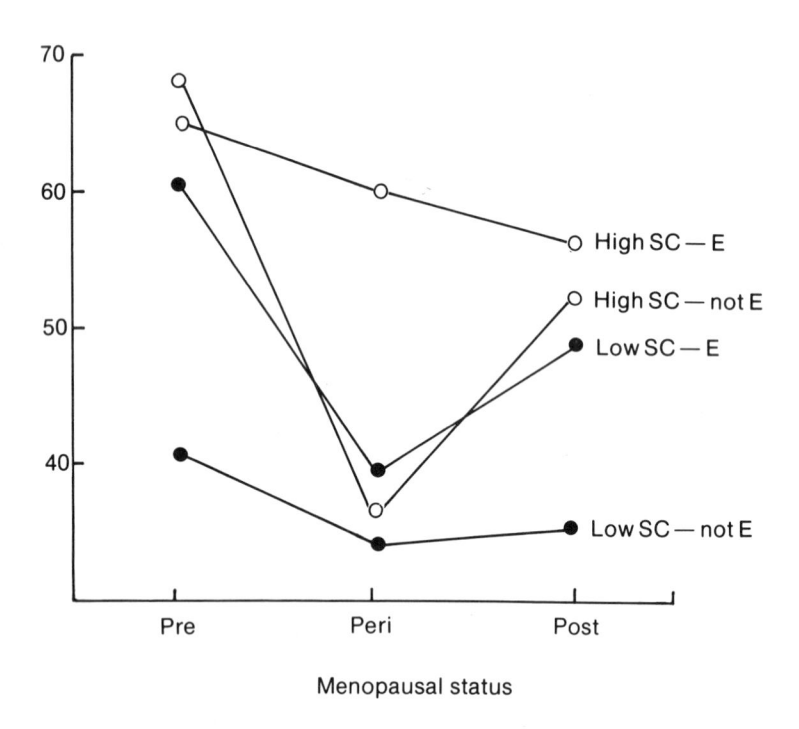

Figure 5.7 Percentage of women showing good subjective adaptation in relation to employment (E) and social class (SC).

(adapted from Severne, 1979)

mainly to a large increase in such symptoms among women of low socioeconomic status, especially if they are working. Once again, the separate treatment of vasomotor and non-vasomotor symptoms is seen to be justified. Not only do the former show a more dramatic increase at the perimenopause, but the lesser increase in the latter is associated with social factors. Vasomotor symptoms, unlike psychological ones, are again shown to be essentially uninfluenced by such factors. In this respect these findings are totally consistent with those of Polit and Larocco (1980), Greene and Cooke (1980) and Campagnoli et al. (1981).

As in the case of symptoms, Severne, in reporting the effect these two sociodemographic factors, social class and employment status, have on the other characteristics of Belgian women, examined their combined effect. Figure 5.7 illustrates the relationship between these two social factors and Subjective Adaptation. As can be seen, at most menopausal stages, women of lower socioeconomic status showed poor Subjective Adaptation, a finding which is consistent with that of the Swiss survey (see Figure 5.3). These findings would also be consistent with the observation made above in reference to that survey, namely, that in general the acceleration effect at the menopause on functions declining with age, is greater among women of low socioeconomic status. Thus, not only do women of low social class function at a lowish level throughout the climacteric, but any exacerbation effect at the time of the menopause tends to be greater in these women. However, as with symptoms this interpretation must be modified in the light of the effect of employment status.

Among women of high social class employment has the effect of preventing any acceleration in the decline of Subjective Adaptation at the perimenopause, but has no such preventive effect among women of low social class (see Figure 5.7). It should be noted that women of lower social class who are not employed have poor levels of Subjective Adaptation throughout the climacteric. A similar but not so marked pattern was found in regards to the association between social class and employment status and normative integration, thereby suggesting that this sort of pattern, at least for this group of women, is unlikely to be an artefact. There is therefore absolutely no acceleration in age related functions at the menopause among women of high socioeconomic status who are employed, the most consistent effect of the latter being to protect such women from undue decline.

Thus, in these paradoxical relationships, being employed seems to *protect* women of higher social class, but has no beneficial effect, and may even be harmful, to thse of lower social class. Severne accounts for this by suggesting that 'it might well be that the combination of a household and a physically demanding job is for many less privileged women too much at that time' (p.108). This observation would complement that made earlier in this section in relation to the studies of Prill (1966) and Polit and Larocco (1980). Namely, that employment is beneficial only if it is

Table 5.8
Sociodemographic Factors and Climacteric Symptoms

Authors	Low Socioeconomic Status	Low Income	Low Education	Not Employed	Part-time Employed	Being Married	Parity, number of children etc.
McKinlay and Jefferys (1974)	0		0	0		0	0
Jaszmann et al. (1969b)		+	+			+	0
Greene and Cooke (1980)	+						
Campagnoli et al. (1981)	+			+			
Prill (1966)				+			
Polit and Larocco (1980)		0	+	+	+	0	0
Holte and Mikkelsen (1982)		+	0	+		0	
Van Keep and Kellerhals (1974, 1975)	+						
Severne (1979)	+			+			

+ = Factor found to be associated with symptom frequency or severity
0 = Factor found not to be so associated

intrinsically rewarding, and not if it is only for the purpose of supplementing the family income, as it is for many working class women.

This statement from Severne (1982) serves as an apt conclusion to this section:

> Our results show that the menopause has a very different impact on the different groups of women considered; groups who are clearly unequipped to cope with changes at this phase of life. In general, the more privileged women, who have greater material and educational facilities and who live in a more stimulating environment with more resources and more possible choices in life, are less prone to the difficulties of the climacteric (p.247).

The outcome of studies investigating the effects of sociodemographic variables on climacteric symptoms is summarised in Table 5.8.

5.4. SUMMARY AND CONCLUSION

We are now in a position to summarise the influence psycho-sociological factors have on women's responses during the climacteric. The following points can be made.

1. A consideration of the seven studies in which the departure or absence of children from the home has been investigated leads to the conclusion that this has very little effect on the symptoms and general wellbeing of the great majority of climacteric women. Of these seven empirical investigations in only one, the IHF Swiss study, was loss of maternal role associated with an elevation of symptoms, and this occurred among *pre*menopausal women only (Table 5.1).
2. The main familial factor which does seem to emerge as being associated with adverse reaction during the climacteric are marital relations. In two of the three studies in which these were examined, more women complaining of marital dissatisfaction reported symptoms than those who had satisfactory marital relations, and this appears to occur throughout the climacteric. The exception to this finding was the study by Crawford and Hooper (1973), which was a particularly poorly designed one. It will also be recalled that one of the factors noted by Hallstrom (1977) as contributing to

declining sexual interest in climacteric women was an unhappy marital situation (see section 4.2).
3. Marital problems are likely to be of a longstanding nature and there are no indications from any of these studies that such problems began during the climacteric. Indeed, the study of Uphold and Susman (1981) and both IHF studies indicate that marital relations are not greatly affected at that time. This suggests that the exacerbation of non-specific symptoms during the climacteric (section 3.2) may, in part at least, be associated with pre-existing psychosocial difficulties.
4. Schneider and Brotherton (1979) also implicate what could be seen to be longstanding problems, such as economic difficulties and problems in early psychological development as contributing to depression in climacteric women. It is unlikely, however, that the depression shown by these women had anything to do with the menopause (see section 4.3) and indeed of the 'stress' factors thought to be particularly associated with the time of the climacteric — the empty nest, loss of reproductive function, ageing parents — none showed any relationship to depression in that study.
5. As far as sociodemographic influences are concerned, it is clear that it is underprivileged women, that is, women of lower socioeconomic status, of low family income and of low educational level, who are likely to experience more numerous and more severe symptoms at the time of the climacteric (Table 5.8).
6. Women who have no occupation outwith the home are by and large more vulnerable, but this effect too is associated with being underprivileged, as employment has a beneficial effect if a woman is of high social class but may have a detrimental effect if she is of low social class. The effect of being employed is further compounded by the fact that to have a beneficial effect, such employment requires to be intrinsically rewarding and perhaps career orientated, something which is less feasible for women of low socioeconomic status.
7. Where a distinction has been made between different types of symptoms, the main effects of sociodemographic factors are on the non-vasomotor symptoms, and in particular psychological ones (Severne, 1979; Greene and Cooke, 1980; Polit and Larocco, 1980; Campagnoli et al., 1981).
8. For the most part sociodemographic factors seem to exercise their effects across all menopausal status groups, that is

throughout the climacteric. There is, however, some evidence from the IHF studies that when psychological symptoms are exacerbated at the menopause, this effect is greater among women of lower socioeconomic status. A similar effect was observed in regard to other social and psychological characteristics, particularly those declining with age, including sexual functioning.

Conclusion

The available evidence indicates that circumstances peculiar to the time of the climacteric, such as the departure of children from home, the loss of the parental and reproductive function are *not* factors which make women to any great degree susceptible to develop symptoms at that time of life. On the contrary, such symptoms appear to be associated more with pre-existing or longstanding difficulties, such as marital dissatisfaction, financial difficulties and problems in early development. Such pre-existing problems may act to heighten the exacerbation of symptoms at the menopause. An alternative way of looking at this is to regard the effect of these problems on symptoms, which in the case of marital problems occur throughout the climacteric, as being accentuated by the event of the menopause. This may be a more appropriate causal mode in cases where marital problems pre-date the climacteric.

Nor is there any support for the commonly held view that preoccupation with, and adverse reactions during the climacteric period of life is a prerogative of middle and upper class women. Indeed the evidence indicates that the reverse is the case, in that it is mainly underprivileged women of low socioeconomic status, low income, low educational level with limited employment prospects, who suffer most at that time. In fact women of higher social class who are employed appear to show little ill effects at all during the climacteric. These demographic factors exercise their influences, as might be expected, mainly on psychological symptoms and functions throughout the climacteric, although their effects may be heightened at time of final menses. In short, the tendency during the climacteric for decline in social or psychological functioning to be accelerated, for already existing problems to be accentuated and for previous difficulties to recur, (noted in the conclusion section of the preceding chapter) is considerably greater among women belonging to socially less privileged groups and those with longstanding psychosocial problems. Again it is factors which *pre-date* the climacteric, rather than psychosocial changes occurring specifically at that time, which are found to determine adverse reactions.

6

Sociocultural Determinants of Women's Responses During the Climacteric

The impression emerging from the two preceding chapters is that much of the adverse reaction shown by women during the climacteric is associated with pre-existing problems — psychological, social, marital, sexual, psychiatric — and that these reactions are in turn mediated by pre-existing psychosocial and sociodemographic factors, moreso than by factors thought to be peculiar to, or occurring particularly at that time of life. In this chapter this theme is developed by considering the extent to which another set of pre-existing factors, namely social attitudes to and expectancies about the menopause, mediate reactions during the climacteric. We have seen, for example, in the study by Dennerstein et al. (1977) how women's preconceptions about sexual difficulties prior to surgical menopause influenced whether or not they actually experienced loss of libido postoperatively (section 4.2). An important determinant therefore, as to how women respond during the climacteric may be the attitudes they have formed to the menopause and their perceptions of its consequences, real or imagined. However, as these consequences and attitudes, like attitudes to any other social phenomenon, are likely to be coloured by the overall cultural milieu of a society, it is of some importance to view these attitudes within the context of the prevailing social mores. In this chapter we shall examine the empirical evidence regarding whether, and if so to what extent, these two major determinants, social attitudes and culture, influence women's responses during the climacteric. In this chapter we shall therefore be adopting what is usually referred to as a 'sociocultural approach' to the climacteric, as described by Brooks-Gunn (1982). For obvious reasons the majority of studies discussed in this chapter have focused on the specific event of the menopause.

6.1. STUDIES OF ATTITUDES TO THE MENOPAUSE

Although the importance of attitudes to the menopause in determining women's responses to that event is frequently stressed in the climacteric literature (see for example relevant chapters in Beard, 1976; Campbell, 1976; van Keep et al., 1979; Haspels and Musaph, 1979 and Voda et al., 1982), as Eisner and Kelly (1980) have pointed out there is in fact a dearth of knowledge in this area. Indeed, in none of the studies to be discussed in this section has there been any attempt to examine systematically the relationship between differing attitudes and women's actual responses at the menopause, either in terms of symptoms or some other outcome measure. Furthermore, in only one study has an attempt been made to look in any detail at the psychological antecedents of attitudes to the menopause. The methods employed in each of the main studies to be reviewed below are summarised in Table 6.1, and it is on the subject of method that we begin.

Table 6.1

Summary of Empirical Studies of Attitudes to the Menopause

Authors	Location	Source of Sample	Size and Age	Measure of Attitude	Factors Associated with Negative Attitude
Neugarten et al. (1963)	Chicago, USA	Mothers of high school pupils	267 21–65	ATM checklist	Younger women
Eisner and Kelly (1980)	Houston, USA	Churches, universities, businesses	393 21–65	ATM checklist	Younger women, women of lower income and education
Dege and Gretzinger (1982)	Detroit, USA	Personal contacts	9 families	ATM checklist, menopause attitude and belief schedule	Younger women, women of low education
International Health Foundation (1969)	Five European countries	Random sample	2000 46–55	13-item questionnaire	Women of low socioeconomic status (Severne, 1979)
Perlmutter and Bart (1982)	Chicago, USA	Religious and civic groups	221 30–70	ATM checklist, menopausal attribution test	Younger women
Maoz et al. (1970)	Israel	General practitioner referrals	55 40–50	10 gain-loss themes	Psychosexual factors (see Table 6.4)

The Attitudes-Toward-Menopause (ATM) Checklist

The first systematic study of women's attitudes to the menopause using a well constructed measure of attitudes, was carried out by Neugarten et al. (1963). The construction of this measure will be described here in some detail as it has become the most frequently used instrument to measure attitudes to the menopause, and as such has been used in several of the studies to follow (see Table 6.1).

The checklist consists of 35 statements, reflecting a wide diversity of opinions, which had originally been collected in the course of a number of exploratory interviews with climacteric women. This checklist was administered to the same group of women who had been subjects in the symptom survey carried out by Neugarten and Kraines (1965) previously described in section 3.2. They consisted of a group of climacteric women, aged 45 to 55 years, 40 of whom were self defined as menopausal, a group of older women aged 56 to 65, all of whom were postmenopausal and two groups of younger women aged 21 to 30 and 31 to 44 years. The responses of these women to each statement, using a four point rating of degree of agreement, were then submitted to a factor analysis (see section 7.4 for a description of this technique). This revealed that the 35 statements could be grouped into seven possible categories, each of which were identified and labelled by the authors as reflecting a different aspect of attitudes towards the menopause.

These categories are shown in Table 6.2 together with an example of a statement from each. Mean percentages of women responding positively to statements within each category for each age group are also shown. As can be seen, major differences emerged between the younger and older age group in three of the categories, with the latter having more optimistic views regarding 'postmenopausal recovery', the 'extent of continuity' and 'control of symptoms'. There was little variation between age groups with regard to any of the four other categories. Women within each group were roughly equally divided as to whether they regarded the menopause with 'negative affect', as a time of 'psychological loss' or as an 'unpredictable event'.

The main finding to emerge from this study therefore, was that younger women, with no direct personal experience of the menopause, had more negative attitudes to that event than did those who were currently experiencing or who had passed through that phase of their lives. It would appear that women may be more apprehensive about the menopause than they need be, and that it does not in retrospect have the negative consequences many fear. Although about half the women, who had experienced the menopause, agreed that the menopause was to some

Table 6.2

Mean Percentages of Women Agreeing to Statements within each Attitude Category for each Age Group

Category of Attitude	Per Cent Agreeing			
	21—30	31—44	45—55	56—65
Negative affect (e.g. menopause is an unpleasant experience)	52	44	53	48
Postmenopausal recovery (e.g. women generally feel better after the menopause)	19	27	60	63
Extent of continuity (e.g. menopause does not really change a woman in any way)	47	59	75	81
Control of symptoms (e.g. women who have trouble are those expecting it)	49	54	75	73
Psychological change (e.g. women often get self-centred at the menopause)	48	45	50	33
Unpredictability (e.g. menopause is a mysterious thing women do not understand)	43	52	56	43
Sexuality (e.g. after the menopause a woman is more interested in sex)	11	30	32	22

Adapted from Neugarten et al. (1963)

extent an unpleasant experience, the majority reported a good recovery from the experience with little or no prolonged effect on their basic personality or life style. A common theme in the literature is that one of women's main concerns at the menopause is the loss of reproductive capacity (see section 5.1). The authors note that little evidence in support of this emerged from this study. Very few women endorsed this view, and in terms of its consequences more were preoccupied with the menopause as a sign of ageing.

In short, this empirical study suggests that the common stereotype of the menopause and its consequences dissipates in the light of experience. The study however, is not without its shortcomings, the main one being the unrepresentative nature of the sample. The sample is biased towards women of upper social class and higher levels of education and it may be that had women from the lower social classes been included, the findings may have been quite different.

Socioeconomic Status and Attitudes

Support for this view comes from a replication of the above study carried out some 17 years later by Eisner and Kelly (1980) using the same Attitudes-Toward-Menopause checklist, but sampling a much wider socioeconomic range of women. The main interest in replicating the study was to determine whether or not there had been any change in women's attitude over time as a result of contemporary feminist thinking. It was predicted that if this thinking had been influential then the stereotype of the menopause would have diminished and that there would be fewer age differences in attitudes. In addition these researchers examined the influence of other variables, such as race, socioeconomic status and level of education on women's attitudes towards the menopause. The sample consisted of 204 white and 189 black women in the age range 21 to 65 years. All were volunteers who were contacted through churches, universities and businesses in the Houston metropolitan area, Texas.

The main findings in brief were that, as in Neugarten's original research, clear age differences emerged. Once again, the younger women (age range 21 to 44) seemed more negative than older menopausal and postmenopausal women in their attitudes to the menopause. While similar differences were found between age groups for both black and white women, the attitudes of black women were, in general, less positive than those of white women. Low income and educational level were also found to be associated with a negative attitude, which perhaps explains the more negative views of black women.

In comparison with women in the earlier study, those in the contemporary study tended to have slightly more positive attitudes towards the menopause. When however, racial groups were compared separately, it emerged that contemporary white women's attitudes had changed in a positive way much more than those of contemporary black women. Although the authors conclude that 'in general there does not seem to be momentous shifts in the direction of more positive attitudes towards the menopause over the last decade and a half' (p.8), it seems likely that among women of higher social class there has been some observable shifts, but what is more interesting is that age differences in attitudes still persist, particularly among women of lower social class.

Additional evidence for the influence of socioeconomic status on attitudes, comes from a study by Dege and Gretzinger (1982), in which the ATM Checklist was also used. This is an unusual study in that not only were the attitudes of women themselves towards the menopause examined, but those of their immediate families were also ascertained. The sample consisted of nine families living in the Detroit area, the criteria for selection being that the woman was living with her husband and had at least one high school aged child. This yielded in all 9 women, 9 husbands and 16 adolescent children. In addition to the ATM Checklist, a Menopause Attitudes and Belief Interview Schedule, constructed by the authors, was administered.

The attitude of the group as a whole tended to be a negative one, with an overall average of 57 per cent negative responses, but this concealed wide intergroup variation. Surprisingly, women themselves had the least negative attitude and children the most. Attitudes, however, tended to be similar within families there being a high level of agreement between women, their husbands and the children. Consistent with the finding of Neugarten et al. (1963) and Eisner and Kelly (1980), younger women had a more negative image of the menopause than did older women. Perhaps the most significant finding of this study however, was the presence of

Table 6.3

Percentage of Positive Responses in Attitude Towards the Menopause

Woman's level of Education	Women	Husbands	Children
High	61	57	45
Low	35	25	35

Adapted from Dege and Gretzinger (1982)

what could be interpreted as a strong social class influence. When families were divided into two groups according to the woman's educational level, those families in which the woman was of a high educational level shared a consistently more positive attitude to the menopause. These differences are shown in Table 6.3.

Family members of women of lower educational status had many more negative attitudes and beliefs about the menopause, thought there was much less communication about these within the family and tended to be less supportive. These families also saw the events occurring around the women at that time of life as involving mainly loss, and discontinuity, resulting in emotional instability. In contrast, those families in which the woman was of high educational attainment viewed the menopause and the events surrounding it as part of a continuous process of life and as a time when 'things were in general getting better'. The authors regard these negative attitudes as primarily determined by social class, being based on a subcultural stereotype of the role and status of the postreproductive women. They also add that 'those who had the most life stress and the least control over it were those who had the most negative attitudes toward menopause' (p.68). Thus the shared attitudes within families appear to reflect a consensus originating from common social class membership and experience.

A similar association between negative attitudes to the menopause and low educational level was observed by Lincoln (1980) in an unpublished doctoral thesis. Severne (1979), in her report on the IHF Swiss survey also briefly noted that although about one third of women expressed a pessimistic view of the climacteric, such women were more often than not of low socioeconomic status and educational level. These class differences she attributed to lack of information and understanding of the menopause among women of low social status.

The International Health Foundation Attitude Survey

In addition to the two major surveys of symptoms, the International Health Foundation had earlier carried out a large scale survey of women's attitudes to the menopause in five European countries in the late sixties (International Health Foundation, 1969). This study was based on personal interviews with 2000 women between the ages 46 to 55 years from each of the countries, Belgium, France, Great Britain, Italy and West Germany. About half these women were postmenopausal, a quarter pre and a quarter perimenopausal. The main instrument for assessing attitudes was a list of 13 statements expressing common views about the menopause to which women were asked to agree or disagree.

In general, attitudes of women to the menopause were fairly positive. The majority of women did not see it as having a major impact on their relations with their spouse, either sexual (55 per cent) or personal (69 per cent), particularly if the couple were happily married (84 per cent), and indeed many women saw positive advantages, particularly with respect to freedom from menstruation (72 per cent) and risk of pregnancy (72 per cent). Most however, did see it as a time of physical upset (69 per cent) and to a lesser degree a time of psychological stress (57 per cent). As far as national variations were concerned there were few marked trends apart from the finding that in general British women had a consistently more optimistic outlook, perhaps reflecting the stoicism of the average British housewife. Although a large scale study, in terms of the number of subjects, this is not a particularly revealing study. Only percentages of women agreeing or disagreeing with the 13 statements are reported for each national group separately, and no attempt was made to examine the antecedents or consequences of particular attitudes.

An Attributional Approach

An interesting approach to the study of attitudes is that of Perlmutter and Bart (1982), who utilise an attributional model as a means of understanding how attitudes may mediate between, on the one hand, the physiological changes, and on the other hand, the psychological responses of women at the time of the menopause. This approach is based on the theory of Schachter (1964), who has demonstrated how individuals rely on situational cues to arrive at a cognitive understanding of poorly understood bodily states. In the context of the menopause these authors suggest that if, for example, the menopause implies ageing to a women, and this is unacceptable to her, then menopausal changes could cue in depression due to the interpretation she makes of her bodily experience. That is, 'the real physiological changes of the menopause are given meaning through a cognitive labelling process that is influenced by psychological and sociocultural elements' (p.183).

Perlmutter (1981) describes an experimental study in which an attributional person-perception format is used to test this hypothesis. The subjects consisted of 221 women between the age of 30 and 70 years living in the Chicago area who were contacted through local religious and civic groups. The assessment instrument was a Menopausal Attribution Test in which the subject reads stories, about which they are later asked questions regarding the main character's mood, personality and the causes of the mood. The mood and menopausal status of this main character naturally vary between stories. A modified version of the Attitudes-Toward-Menopause Checklist of Neugarten et al. (1963) and information relating to sociodemographic variables were also included in the research protocol.

In brief, the results of this study showed that subjects reported a slightly positive overall attitude towards the menopause, but they also believed that the menopause was associated with negative but not positive moods. In general, sociodemographic variables were found not to be related to attitudes but older subjects and those who were postmenopausal tended to have more positive attitudes than younger women. The latter is of course consistent with the findings of Neugarten et al. (1963), Eisner and Kelly (1980) and Dege and Gretzinger (1982). The former finding which is inconsistent with other work could be due to the sample being biased towards the middle to upper social classes, thereby giving a narrow socioeconomic range.

On the basis of this model and her findings, Perlmutter suggests that endocrine changes may lead to alterations in physiological arousal which produces a potentiation of both positive and negative moods. Women then apply the available cognitive labels to these experiences, and hold the menopause responsible for negative affect but look to other factors, such as situational events to explain positive moods, thus reinforcing the general stereotype of the menopause. This is an interesting and novel approach to the linking of the physical and psychic aspects of the menopause and as such is worthy of further investigation.

Psychosexual Factors and Attitudes

The only empirical study in which any attempt has been made to investigate possible psychological antecedents of attitudes to the menopause is that by Maoz et al. (1970). The study was carried out on a population of women of mixed ethnic origin living in the state of Israel. The authors began with the hypothesis that women who had coped in a satisfactory way with other psychosexual experiences would tend to have a more positive attitude to the menopause than those who had not. More specifically they predicted that there would be a relationship between response to the menopause and the nature and quality of, for example, experiences in adolescence, pregnancy, childbirth, marriage and sexual relations.

The data reported in this paper were based on a series of individual semistructured psychiatric interviews. The sample consisted of 55 married women within the age range 40 to 55 years, most of whom were referred to the research team by general practitioners or nurses. Most of the women were described as being generally physically healthy, but 11, that is 20 per cent, were psychiatric patients known to be suffering from 'chronic emotional and psychosomatic disorders'. In no respect therefore can the group be considered a random sample and in fact the indications are that if anything subjects were somewhat atypical. Thirty of the women were Jewish of European origin, and 17 Jewish of Afro-Asian origin, the remaining 8 being Israeli Arabs. Using a criteria based on a mixture of last menstrual period and presence of vasomotor symptoms, 17 women were classified as pre, 23 as peri and 11 as postmenopausal. However, in the analysis the group is treated as a whole, regardless of menopausal status.

Women's attitude to the menopause was determined in terms of ten 'themes', consisting of consequences of the menopause. Three of these consequences were 'gains', that is being free from menstruation, freedom from pregnancy and a non-specific sense of liberation. The other seven themes consisted of 'losses'. These were loss of fertility, health and femininity, the onset of old age, the dangers of emotional or somatic disturbance and a general feeling that 'it had come too soon'. On this basis 18 women were classified as having a positive, and 27 as having a negative attitude, leaving 6 who could not be easily classified. Data were presented showing the relationship between the dependent variable — attitude to the menopause — and ten other variables including the items pertaining to psychosexual history.

For the group as a whole the salient findings were as follows. More women with a *negative* attitude to the menopause had received prior information about the menarche, recollected having had a pleasant or normal adolescence, had a positive attitude to menstruation or regarded it as a 'natural' process, had a desire to have more children, but had fertility problems. Data relating to these findings are summarised in Table 6.4. These findings clearly fail to support the authors' hypothesis that women who had coped successfully with previous psychosexual experiences would do similarly in respect to the menopause. Indeed, if anything, the reverse is the case.

Although the authors state that they are unable to say 'what are the decisive factors in determining responses of women to the climacterium' (p.39), there does seem to be a common theme running through these psychosexual experiences which is related to reproductive function and how this is evaluated by some women. It would appear that among this sample of women there are some who have highly valued their reproductive function and consequently family life. They have a positive attitude to menstruation, seeing it as a natural process, and have been adequately informed about it, presumably by their parents, and have had a normal adolescence. They have a desire for more children, but some have had fertility problems. Such women are unlikely to welcome the menopause for obvious reasons. Thus, it is a small group of women who have had, or who have wanted, a satisfactory reproductive life, who come out in this study as being the most negative in their attitude to the menopause.

Table 6.4

*Attitude to the Menopause of Israeli Women
in Relation to earlier Psychosexual Experience*

	Attitude	
	Positive	Negative
Attitude to menstruation		
Postive	5	18
Negative	6	6
Information about menarche		
Prior information	2	8
No prior information	11	8
Adolescence		
Happy	3	12
Unhappy	7	7
Pregnancy and childbirth		
No difficulties	8	11
Some difficulties	10	11
Fertility problems	0	5
Desire for more children		
Yes	0	13
No	11	10

Adapted from Maoz et al. (1970)

This conclusion however, must be tempered in the light of a number of inadequacies in the design of the study. In addition to being unrepesentative of the general population, from which it was chosen, there being a high degree of known psychopathology in the group, the sample was unduly small, and no inferential tests were carried out. Probably a more serious flaw in the design is a confounding of the method of measuring attitude to the menopause and the method of measuring the psychosexual variables. It is not surprising that a variable, such as a desire to have more children is associated with a negative attitude to the menopause when one of the items used to determine a negative attitude is concern over loss of fertility. A similar comment can be made regarding the relationship between a positive attitude to menstruation and a negative attitude to the menopause, when freedom from menstruation is used to classify women as having a positive attitude to the menopause. This is clearly tautologous since the dependent variable — attitude to menopause — is being measured in terms of some of the independent variables. This method of assessing attitudes to menopause is therefore an unsatisfactory one and inferior to that developed by Neugarten et al. (1963).

The finding that concern about loss of reproductive function is related to negative attitudes to the menopause is contrary to the finding of Neugarten et al. (1963) in the first study reviewed in this section. However, the group of women in the Israeli study were of mixed ethnic origin, and as we shall see in the next section such concerns tend to be determined by cultural factors. The outcome of empirical studies of attitudes to the menopause are summarised in the last column of Table 6.1.

6.2. CULTURAL VARIATION

How individuals conceptualise and react to a psychosocial event or change is obviously influenced by the prevailing customs, mores and values of the society within which they find themselves — what anthropologists refer to as the 'culture' of the society. There seems little reason to doubt that attitudes to, and behaviour at the menopause will also be similarly influenced by the prevailing cultural milieu and the particular significance attached to that event within the society (Brooks-Gunn, 1982). Evidence for wide variation in this comes from a review by Griffen (1977) of crosscultural differences in changes in behaviour among women at the time of the menopause. This review was based on an examination of the Human Relations Area Files, a catalogue of reports by anthropologists who have carried out fieldwork in various societies. At the time of the review some 267 different cultures were indexed on the File.

Of these 267 cultures, only 35 contained any entry relevant to behavioural change at or after the climacteric. In ten of these it was noted that these changes were similar for both men and women, that is, the changes were not peculiar to women. For a further eight cultures it was specifically noted that no behaviour change occurred at all among postmenopausal women. For the remaining 17 cultures, Griffen classified the behaviour change into four categories. First, there were cultures within which women were expected to begin to withdraw from previous social activities. Secondly, in two cultures, both African, the menopause was regarded as an actual illness with the appropriate accompanying 'illness behaviour'. Thirdly, there were several other cultures in which the behaviour of postmenopausal women changed in the direction of greater freedom, and finally, there were a few, mostly North American, in which the menopause signalled access to increased social and supernatural powers. On the basis of this, albeit, scanty information, Griffen concluded that these files 'seem to demonstrate that behaviour proper to the role of the elderly female is shaped by culture, as are all sex and age-linked roles' (p.54). It is also clear from these files, sparse though they may be, that there is a great diversity among societies as to how the menopause is viewed and certainly no general rule for the menopause to be regarded either in a negative or positive fashion in other cultures.

In the material examined by Griffen, most of the references to social and behavioural change at the menopause were reported incidently to other purposes and observations, and that in the case of only 13 per cent of the records. A number of systematic studies, however, have been carried out in which authors have specifically set out to examine attitudes and reactions to the menopause, in an empirical way among women of different ethnic origin, both within and across societies. We begin the review of these studies, which are listed in Table 6.5, by returning to one discussed at the end of the previous section, that by Maoz et al. (1970).

Cultural Variation in Attitude to the Menopause

The study by Maoz et al. (1970) is in fact the first of a number of reports coming from this Israeli research group on cultural influences during the climacteric. As the authors point out, because of the multi-ethnic character of the population, Israel offers a rich opportunity for comparative crosscultural studies. It will be recalled that in this study the sample investigated consisted of a group of women of mixed ethnic origin.

Differences were noted in several respects between women of European and those of Oriental-Arab origin. Some 60 per cent of the former, for example, had a negative attitude to the menopause as against 43 per cent of the latter, in terms of the 'gain-loss' criteria used to assess attitude in this study. There were also differences between the two ethnic groups in regard to the associations between negative attitudes and the various psychosexual factors (for these see Table 6.4). Among European women most of these factors were associated to a slight degree with a negative attitude, whereas among Oriental-Arab women a negative attitude was related only, but to a strong degree, to a desire to have more

Table 6.5
Summary of Cross Cultural Studies of Women's Responses during the Climacteric

Authors	Country	Ethnic Groups Studied	Main Findings
Maoz et al. (1970)	Israel	Jewish women of European origin, Orienti-Arab women	More Europeans had negative attitudes.
Dowtry et al. (1970)	Israel	Jewish women of European and Afro-Asian origin, Arab women	Europeans more concerned with psychological and social consequences; others more with physical and biological.
Flint and Garcia (1979)	USA	Jewish women, Cuban immigrants	Jewish women more concerned with psychological consequences; Cubans more with loss of reproductive function.
Flint (1979)	India	Rajput women	Symptoms infrequent, attitudes positive.
Moore (1981)	Zimbabwe	Mashona women	Symptoms highly common.
Maoz et al. (1977, 1978)	Israel	Jewish women of European, Turkish, Persian, North African origin; Arab women	Ethnic groups in transitional phase had more symptoms and negative attitudes.
Wright (1981, 1982)	USA	Navajo Indian women	Traditional women report more symptoms than modernised women, former influenced by health and economic factors, latter by social and psychological ones.
Davis (1982)	Canada	Newfoundland women	Symptoms and negative attitudes widespread.
Kearns (1982)	USA	Papago Indian women	Negative attitudes influenced by traditional values, adverse effects of rapid acculturation.

children and a positive view of menstruation. Thus, from the outset, it appears that not only may there be cultural variation in the extent of negative attitudes to the menopause, but the reasons for holding negative attitudes may vary considerably from one culture to another.

This theme was further developed in a second paper from the Israeli group, by Dowtry et al. (1970), in which the reasons different ethnic groups give for holding negative attitudes were discussed in further detail, on the basis of the ten 'themes' or consequences (that is, the gain-loss criteria) described in the previous paper. The three ethnic group, Jewish women of European origin, Jewish women of Afro-Asian origin and Arab women, were considered as representing three points on a continuum from modernity to traditionalism. At one end, women of European origin had the cultural background of an industrial urban Western society, at the other, Arab women lived in a traditional village setting, while Jewish women from North Africa and Asia, many of whom had come from cities in those regions, were considered as being in an intermediate cultural stage. Perceived consequences of the menopause were found to differ between these three groups.

Women of European origin differed from the other two more traditional groups in regard to the *saliency* of the menopause, assessed in terms of the actual degree of severity of consequences. For European women the menopause seemed a less salient or significant event than for the others. Despite this it was also found that European women were much less *uniform* in their choice of consequences, no doubt reflecting the greater plurality of Western industrialised societies as against North African and Arab ones. In regard to the *content* of themes, all three ethnic groups differed as to which consequences were considered important.

Regarding content, women of European origin were less concerned about the physical consequences of the menopause than they were about the concomitant changes relating to personality, the family and their social situation. Both Afro-Asian Jewish and Arab women, on the other hand, emphasised the biological consequences, but whereas the Arab women welcomed the cessation of menses but not the cessation of childbirth, for the Afro-Asian women this was reversed. The authors conclude that the women's perception of the menopause is closely related to her particular cultural role, one of the key features of which is the centrality of the child bearing function to this role. There is a shift along the traditional-modern continuum in this respect from the Arab women, for whom child bearing is still an important function, to the Afro-Asian women, in an intermediate phase, for whom child bearing is less important, but they are still preoccupied by some of the biological consequences of the menopause. For the European woman her relative lack of concern with biological sequelae of the menopause means that she focuses attention more on potential psychological and social changes. Thus, according to these authors, women at different points in the traditional-modern continuum highlight those consequences at the climacteric which result in significant changes in their social role and status. As shall be seen this is a consistent theme in crosscultural studies of the climacteric.

Another comparative study illustrating how negative attitudes towards the menopause may be held for different reasons by different ethnic groups is one carried out in the State of New Jersey in the United States by Flint and Garcia (1979). These authors compared the attitudes to the menopause of two ethnically different groups, consisting of 40 middle class Jewish women and 34 Cuban women, most from professional backgrounds, living in that state. Both groups were of a similar socioeconomic level. However, Jewish women had lived in the United States all their lives, whereas all Cuban women had been born in Cuba, and still identified with Spanish culture, as well as the Cuban subculture. The study focused on those women having negative attitudes to the menopause and their reasons for holding such attitudes.

In brief, negative attitudes, when they existed among Jewish women, were found to be due to the menopause symbolising ageing and behavioural decline. This attitude, according to Flint (1979), reflects the prevailing cultural norm in the United States. Among Cuban women, despite being of a professional background, negative attitudes to the menopause were more common and were based mainly on the menopause as ending their reproductive capacity. This was also thought to be associated with guilt over sexual relations when procreation is no longer possible. This traditional attitude to sex was also reflected in the reluctance of Cuban women to respond in the study to questions about their sexual attitudes and behaviour. The point to be made here is that, as in the studies by the Israeli workers, negative attitudes to the menopause may have an entirely different basis within societies of mixed ethnic origins, depending on the subcultural mores, and other values such as, as in this case, religiously based beliefs.

Role and Status

In the course of an earlier examination of the Human Relations Area Files, which predated that of Griffen (1977), Bart (1969) noted that 'certain structural arrangements and cultural values' were associated with women's status after the childbearing years. She observed that a strong tie to family of origin and kin, rather than a strong marital tie, an extended family system rather than a nuclear one, an institutionalised grandmother role rather than no formal role, a defined mother-in-law role and residence patterns keeping one close to the family of origin, all seemed to be associated with improved status in middle age. Bart suggested that 'even if there are physiological stresses at this time, they are well buffered structurally in kinship-dominated societies' (in Bart and Grossman, 1978, p.345). It is obvious that the foregoing are all features of highly traditional societies.

Nevertheless, it would be misleading to assume that traditionalism per se is associated with improved status in middle life and consequently with positive response at the climacteric. This can be demonstrated by comparing the findings of the next two studies, both of traditional societies, in one of which the consequences of the menopause is to enhance and in the other to diminish social status, these outcomes being due to the influence of cultural mores peculiar to the particular society.

The first of these studies (Flint, 1975; 1979) comes from India and consists of a survey of the attitudes to the menopause of Rajput women, a caste residing within the Indian states of Rajasthan and Himachal Pradesh. This group of women were chosen as members of this caste are large land owners and the women well nourished in comparison to other populations in India. When asked about problems associated with the menopause few women reported any, other than the change in the menstrual cycle. Few reported depression, headaches or any of the classical symptoms associated with the climacteric. Indeed, many women informed the author that they were looking forward to this stage in their lives, if they had not yet reached it, and if they had, they were entirely positive about the event.

The explanation of this lies, of course, in the culturally determined changes in the woman's social role and status heralded by the menopause in that particular culture. In Rajasthan, Rajput women live in purdah prior to the menopause. In Himachal Pradesh women, while not in purdah, are not allowed to be in the company of men other than their husbands, and before marriage their fathers. With the attainment of the menopause, these women, who had been restricted in many of their activities due to cultural taboos, now experience a change in status as well as role. In Rajasthan, Rajput women are released from purdah and in Himachal Pradesh they can now freely consort with other men. By becoming menopausal the status of these women is now more elevated than it was while they were able to bear children.

Much has been made of this study by, for example, Kaufert (1982) and Wilbush (1982) as illustrating how the menopause need not only have no adverse social consequences but may indeed result in a marked *increase* in a woman's social status. It could of course be argued that the change in status of postmenopausal Rajput women must be seen relative to their previous low status. The social taboos on premenopausal women are, in fact, due to their being considered unclean and contaminated while still capable of menstruating and bearing children. In Rajput society therefore, the cessation of menses removes a social stigma and with it certain social constraints. Such a change of status is therefore essentially a negative phenomenon and this may hold in other societies in which a putative elevation of status is said to occur at the climacteric.

In contrast to this study, one by Moore (1981) from Africa demonstrates that the coming of the menopause can have an unquivocably disastrous effect on a woman's position in a traditional society. The sample consisted of 50 randomly selected women belonging to the Mashona group of tribes living in the vicinity of a rural township in South East Zimbabwe. All women were more than one and less than ten years past the date of their last menstrual cycle and were well nourished and in good general health. Symptoms were assessed by means of a questionnaire and were classified as autonomic (hot flushes, sweats, palpitations, dyspepsia), metabolic (dyspareunia, vaginal dryness, joint pains etc.) or psychogenic (depression, anxiety, irritability, etc.).

Forty three per cent of the group were found to be experiencing autonomic symptoms, 52 per cent metabolic and 58 per cent psychogenic symptoms. Unlike for example Rajput women, this general population of Mashona women had very high levels of symptomatology not, according to the author, dissimilar to the recorded incidence of symptoms among *clinical* populations of climacteric women in Western societies. The author attributes this to the fact that in a polygamous society, such as the Mashona, the status of postmenopausal women is a tenuous one. Once a woman has completed her child bearing role she is at the risk of having her marriage dissolved by her husband and of being replaced by a younger, fertile woman. She may therefore face loneliness and destitution, unless she has the protection and support of her adult children. The lesson from this study is that, as Moore succinctly puts it, it provides 'no support for the popularly expressed opinion that the climacteric syndrome is restricted to affluent societies in which healthy middle aged women have the time to over react to the loss of youth and to the prospect of coming old age' (p.29).

Role and Cultural Stability

The hypothesis regarding the association between traditionalism, high status and role stability and positive response at the menopause must be further modified and expanded in the light of a later and much larger scale study by the Israeli researchers (Maoz et al., 1977), in which the population studied consisted of 1148 women living in Israel, of five different ethnic origins. In this study, in addition to attitudes, symptomatology of the five groups was compared. As in the earlier study by Maoz et al. (1970), one group was of Central European origin and represented a modernised, urban, literate group. At the other extreme were again Arab women living in a traditional village setting. Between these two extremes were three other groups, described as being at different transitional stages in the modern-traditional continuum. These consisted of Jewish women of Turkish origin, who were closer culturally to the Central Europeans but of lower socioeconomic status, then Jewish women of North African origin, and lastly Jewish women of Persian origin, who were closer culturally and socioeconomically to the Arab women.

Measures of both symptoms and attitudes were obtained for women in all five ethnic groups. Symptoms were assessed by means of the checklist used by Neugarten and Kraines (1965). Each symptom was scored according to severity on a 1 to 3 basis and total scores for each of the subgroup of symptoms — somatic, psychosomatic and psychological — were calculated. Attitudes to the menopause were assessed by means of a list of 23 statements to which the woman was asked to agree or disagree. This list was based on the findings of the earlier study by Maoz et al. (1970), and opinions were categorised into five different areas of concern. These were cessation of fertility, physical health, emotional health, social-personal changes and changes in husband-wife relations. The authors predicted that there would be a linear relationship between the modern-traditional continuum and women's attitudes and symptoms. This however was not the case, the relationship being more a curvilinear one.

In regard first to attitudes, both Jewish women of Central European origin and Arab women had in general more positive attitudes to the menopause, the three ethnic groups in the transitional phase viewing the consequences of the menopause in more negative terms. Again, however, when European Jewish women and Arab women did express negative attitudes the former were more concerned with emotional consequences and the latter with biological effects. In the case of symptoms, the main finding was that there were no significant differences between groups in somatic symptoms, but Jews of European origin and Arab women had fewer psychosomatic and psychological symptoms than did the other three groups, thereby reflecting the group differences in attitudes. The results in regard to symptoms are summarised in Table 6.6. There, somatic symptoms, and in particular vasomotor symptoms, can be seen to be remarkably stable across the five cultural groups, confirming, according to the authors 'that only the vasomotor symptoms are definitely hormone-related' (p.75).

Table 6.6
Mean Symptom Scores of five Ethnic Groups in Israel

Type of Symptom	Modern-Traditional Continuum				
	European	Turkish	N. African	Persian	Arab
Somatic	6.1	6.3	7.0	7.1	7.2
Psychosomatic	4.1	4.8	5.2	5.6	4.5
Psychological	6.8	8.5	8.4	9.2	8.1

Adapted from Maoz et al. (1977)

In effect the authors' expectation of a linear relationship between responses to the climacteric and the modern-traditional continuum was not upheld, in that it was Arab women at one end of the continuum who seemed to have the most positive view of the climacteric, and European women at the other end, who seemed least concerned, it being the transitional groups which had the most negative attitudes and most complaints. The authors interpret this as indicating that it is not so much the content of a particular ethnic group's culture which matters, as the *stability* of the sociocultural milieu.

In a second paper from the same study, Maoz et al. (1978) went onto examine symptoms in relation to employment status within each of these five ethnic groups. It will be recalled (section 5.3) that in his study of German women, Prill (1977) found that women who had professional careers suffered less during the climacteric than those who did not. However, in the IHF Belgian survey, Severne (1979) had found that working outwith the home helped only those women of higher social class. The Israeli group considered that the protective nature of work might also vary from one culture to another. That is, they anticipated that the influence of the modern-traditional factor would be similar to that of social class in that women from modern ethnic groups would benefit from such employment, whereas those from more traditional cultural backgrounds would not. In the event this proved to be only partly true.

Modern women, represented by Jews of European origin, did indeed suffer less at the climacteric if they worked, thereby confirming Severne's findings with Belgian women. But this also held for two of the more traditional groups — the Arab women and Jewish women from North Africa. Jewish women of Persian origin, on the other hand, generally did not benefit if they worked outside the home. This indeed was the only traditional group to follow the expected pattern, as women of Turkish origin showed no consistent pattern.

Thus the protective function of work outwith the home was not entirely associated with the modern-traditional continuum. Nor was it related to socioeconomic status, as reported in the IHF Belgian study. Both the North African and Persian Jewish women belong to the same low socioeconomic class, but the effect of work on these two groups of women was quite different. The authors conclude therefore that other health, ethnic and social factors peculiar to a particular culture must be contributing to these variations.

Applying Bart's hypothesis regarding the protective nature of kinship dominated societies to that of the Israeli researchers regarding the importance of the stability of the sociocultural milieu, it seems likely that postmenopausal women living in societies at the traditional end of the continuum are protected from some of the consequences of that time because of the availability within kinship dominated societies of alternative social roles, some of which are useful and carry high status. Problems arise as the tightly knit kinship structure breaks down under the impact of modernisation. Such roles become fragmented, and may well disappear until stability returns at a certain level of modernisation, and new roles established. Furthermore, as not all groups of women within a changing society pass through this transitional phase at the same rate, it may be that this accounts for the wide variation in attitudes and responses within modern and pluralistic societies, as demonstrated in section 5.3. Relevant to this point are the findings of an anthropological field study by Wright (1981a), of an Indian tribal group in the United States, in which the symptoms of a group of traditional women were compared with a more modernised group from the same tribe, the latter being described as 'acculturated' by the author.

The subjects consisted of 66 middle aged Navajo women, who were interviewed in the course of an anthropological field work study of this tribe living on reservations in north eastern Arizona. Symptoms were elicited in two ways. First by means of an open ended question about 'bodily changes' in the time since their periods stopped, and secondly by means of a checklist of 16 symptoms. These were subdivided into vasomotor, physical and psychological symptoms. Virtually all respondents reported that there had been no 'bodily changes' in answer to the open ended question, but when asked if they experienced symptoms on the checklist, most responded affirmatively. According to the author, symptom prevalence among the Navajo is very similar to that reported for Western women, when the conventional checklist method is used. Wright goes on to suggest that this finding is due to the fact that Navajo women have an 'unelaborated concept' of the menopause and do not associate any symptoms with the cessation of menses. She concludes that the reporting of such symptoms as menopausal, is influenced by culturally specific expectations and beliefs about the relationship of these complaints to the menopause.

Another finding was that 'traditional' Navajo women, that is those who were uneducated, spoke no English, lived in rural areas and were not in paid employment, reported more of all three types of symptoms than did those who were 'acculturated'. The latter held wage paying jobs, had completed high school and lived in towns on the reservation. These differences in symptoms, shown in Table 6.7, reflect in part the high value placed on the child bearing role of women within traditional Navajo

Table 6.7

Mean Number of Symptoms Reported by Navajo Women

Type of Symptom	Traditional	Acculturated (modernised)
Vasomotor	1.50	1.07
Physical	4.03	3.11
Psychological	2.50	1.86

Adapted from Wright (1981a)

culture (Wright, 1981b). It could also imply, if the hypothesis of the Israeli workers is correct regarding the importance of the stability of a culture, that it is the 'traditional' Navajo women who are in a less stable cultural environment than those who have been 'acculturated' or modernised. Clearly, one of the problems here is of determining when a society, or a group within a society, is passing through a transitional or unstable social phase, a problem which is highlighted in the next study.

The view that role stability and high status act to protect women during the climacteric has been challenged by Davis (1982) on the basis of an anthropological study of 38 women living in a Newfoundland fishing village. In this 'traditional community' the author, using Bart's criteria (Bart, 1969), claims that women have high status, self-esteem and an active and satisfying social role, which continues throughout middle life. Despite this it was found that negative attitudes towards the menopause, as measured by the Neugarten ATM checklist (Neugarten et al., 1963), were extremely pronounced among these women, and that physical and psychological symptoms were commonly associated with the menopause and experienced by the majority of women aged 45 to 55 years. Indeed, as can be seen from Table 6.8, the ATM checklist categories of 'negative affect', 'psychological' loss and 'unpredictability' were all considerably greater among these women at all ages, than those in the original United States sample of urban women.

The author therefore concluded that there is no necessary link between role and status and the nature of women's reactions during the climacteric and that 'the biological changes of the perimenopause may elicit a common negative response cross-culturally regardless of women's status' (p.216). While the author provides a complicated cultural account as to how women in this community conceptualise the menopausal experience, based on 'local notions of blood and nerves', this does not fully explain why negative attitudes to the menopause among these women are so widespread, much moreso than among urban American women. One possible explanation is that this is in fact a society in transition, as it is clear from the author's account that increased communications, in the form of roads, have opened up this community to the influences of the outside world. Furthermore, it is difficult to reconcile this putative idyllic community with the author's observation that 'the two major factors held to weaken nerves in women are worry over husband while at sea and the chronic stress of hard work and poverty' (p.213). This last point conveniently leads to the final topic in this section.

Cultural and Economic Deprivation

A factor which is often overlooked is that modernity often brings with it physical and economic benefits and it could be argued that these, as much as role and status factors, may, to use Bart's expression, 'buffer' women from the stresses and strains of the climacteric period. Some support for

Table 6.8
Percentages of Women Showing Negative Responses for three Attitude Categories

| | 35—44 years || 45—55 years || 56—65 years ||
	USA	Newfoundland	USA	Newfoundland	USA	Newfoundland
Negative effect	40	87	52	74	44	90
Psychological loss	40	57	46	58	23	80
Unpredictability	51	70	56	65	43	80

Adapted from Davis (1983)

this view comes in a second paper by Wright (1982) from the study of Navajo women, in which the author highlights the effect social deprivation and physically arduous conditions of life may have on women during the climacteric.

In this account Wright reports on the association between symptoms and certain 'potentially relevant cultural variables'. These variables are similar to those already discussed in other parts of this volume and included the empty nest (number of children at home); the availability of postmenopausal roles (care of grandchildren, ceremonial roles); social integration (proximity of relatives, frequency of visiting); attitudes toward menopause (expectation of changes, evaluation of menopause). These variables together with a number of others (evaluation of health, economic rating, education) were then examined in relation to symptoms, using a multiple regression analysis. This allowed the author to evaluate the contribution of one variable to the variability observed in the dependent variable, while other factors were held constant, and 'to reveal structural relationships between both dependent and independent variables'.

The results of this complex analysis can be summarised briefly as the most striking and relevant findings from the standpoint of this review were the clear differences between the two subgroups of women. In the 'acculturated' sample (i.e. modernised women), attitudes towards the menopause consistently related to symptoms, especially psychological ones, with social integration and postmenopausal roles having the next highest association. In the case of the 'traditional' women, concern about health was the best predictor of symptom reporting, particularly those of a physical nature, and economic rating also made a significant contribution in this group. The absence of any contribution from the empty nest situation in either group should be noted. Thus, for acculturated women the factors associated with symptom severity were mostly of a psychological and social nature, whereas for traditional women health and economic factors had the greatest influence.

The author naturally interprets these differing patterns of relationships in terms of the different quality of life of these two groups of women. She writes:

> It is little wonder that economically disadvantaged 'traditional' women and those in ill health suffer the most from menopausal symptoms and that 'traditional' women as a group tend to suffer more from physical complaints ...... Physical demands are apparently minimal and stress is manifested psychologically for the 'acculturated' sample, in terms of both type of factors which influence symptom experience and type of symptoms most affected (p.96).

This tendency for traditional women to emphasise physical and for modern to emphasise psychological change at the menopause is of course reminiscent of the findings of Dowtry et al. (1970).

Another anthropological study of a North American Indian tribal group which implicates physical and social deprivation in the way women respond during the climacteric, is a study by Kearns (1982) of Papago women. The subjects consisted of 100 female members of this tribe living in a reservation in the state of Arizona. From the author's description this seems to be an unusually deprived social group, having a high suicide rate, excessive alcohol abuse, family disorganisation and suffering generally from the effects of rapid acculturation. Among these women there was a high degree of ignorance or incorrect knowledge about the menopause, towards which negative attitudes were widespread. These were largely governed by traditional values and practices, and as in many traditional societies the inability to have more children featured as a major factor in shaping negative attitudes.

However, the author notes that under the impact of the external culture these traditional attitudes appear to be weakening among the younger generation of women of the tribe. Although a limited study, as no comparative data is provided, these observations are of interest in that they demonstrate once again the adverse effects rapid acculturation may have on climacteric women in the context of social and physical deprivation. A summary of the outcome of studies discussed in this section can be found in Table 6.5.

6.3. SUMMARY AND CONCLUSION

On the basis of the foregoing account of the empirical research, it would seem that the suggestion made in the introduction to this chapter regarding the importance of attitudes and sociocultural factors in influencing women's responses during the climacteric has been substantiated by the empirical evidence, thereby allowing us to arrive at some tentative pointers as to how such factors operate.

1. The main trend running through the studies of attitudes is that although some women in Western societies do have an overall negative image of the menopause and its consequences, this is not as widespread nor as marked as has been thought,

and indeed many of its consequences are viewed in a positive fashion.

2. Where a negative attitude does exist it appears to be based in part on a *stereotype* of the menopause, since it is found to be stronger in younger than older women. Among women with actual experience of the event these negative attitudes decline. Hence the use of the word stereotype, meaning those elements of a concept based on a fixed or preconceived notion, not derived from immediate experience.

3. A major influence on attitude to the menopause is again social class, with women of lower socioeconomic status, income and education having more negative expectations (see Table 6.1). This of course is consistent with the adverse effects sociodemographic factors have on symptoms and other functions during the climacteric (section 5.3), and is presumably one of the ways these effects are mediated.

4. There appears to have been some change in attitudes to the menopause in the direction of a less negative one, in the last two decades or so. This has largely occurred among women from higher socioeconomic groups. Among women of less privileged status, the negative image has tended to persist, although even among those women there is now greater diversity in attitude. This may be due to the greater availability of information about the menopause, greater social mobility and the erosion of traditional working class attitudes.

5. Another factor which has been found to be associated with a negative attitude to the menopause is the extent to which a woman has valued her reproductive role and regards the menopause adversely for this reason. This of course may be a culturally based phenomenon and there is good reason to suppose that there is wide variation between different societies in this respect.

6. Not only does the extent of negative attitudes to the menopause vary from one culture to another but the reasons underlying such attitudes vary considerably. These reasons are invariably related to the social consequences of the menopause in a particular society, and how these consequences affect women's role and status.

7. There is a trend in more modern societies for these reasons to be less uniform than in traditional ones. In the former they are related more to a variety of putative social and psychological consequences of the menopause, but in the latter are confined

more to the direct biological and physical consequences of that event.
8. In highly traditional societies the inevitable effect of the menopause on reproductive functioning is often obviated by the availability of alternative social roles, particularly in those societies having strong kinship and family bonds. There is little justification, however, for the view that adverse reactions during the climacteric are a feature unique to modern industrialised societies and that the effect of the climacteric on women in traditional societies is relatively benign.
9. Indeed, a more important factor in this respect is the stage a society is at in the transition between a traditional and modern one. In those societies still in a transitional phase, or in the process of rapid acculturation, attitudes to the menopause and reactions during the climacteric may be more adverse than those of women in more culturally stable modern or traditional societies. This suggests that it is women with a well defined or significant postmenopausal social role, whether it be a modern or traditional one, who are least affected during the climacteric.
10. This is not, however, a universal phenomenon and wide variation occurs in attitudes and responses both within modern societies and between highly traditional ones. Nor is the detrimental effect of work on women of low socioeconomic status a universal phenomenon. The idiosyncratic mores of a culture or subculture, religious beliefs, the speed and impact of modernisation and the presence of physical, social and economic hardship, are all further factors contributing to heterogeneity in response.

Conclusion

In the preceding chapter the profound effect of low socioeconomic status in determining adverse reactions of women during the climacteric was clearly demonstrated. This effect has now been shown to be mediated by the consistently negative attitudes such women hold to the menopause. Moreover, although attitudes to the menopause have been changing among women in general over the last two decades, they are doing so much less rapidly among less privileged women. Such attitudes are, of course, very much rooted in traditional classed based concepts of the female role. While these negative attitudes may at times merely reflect a preconceived idea of, or a cultural stereotype of the menopause, in many instances they are based on the real and direct social consequences of becoming menopausal, particularly in those traditional groups or societies in which child bearing and rearing is seen as a primary function of women. In the latter the consequences of the menopause tend to be regarded as physical and biological, whereas in more modern societies they tend to be social and psychological.

However, from a cultural standpoint, it would seem that on occasions it is women who are living in a transitional society, that is, one in the process of altering from a traditional to a modern social structure, who are the most vulnerable. This is possibly because women living in such changing societies have less well defined and significant postmenopausal social roles. One must be wary, however, that the apparent enhancement in social roles among postmenopausal women in some stable traditional societies is not illusory and merely reflects a relative decrease of stigma or social constraints associated with childbirth and menstruation. Certainly, there are no reasons for assuming that the effects of the climacteric on women living in non-industrialised societies is a benign one, nor in the words of one authority that such women are 'largely symptom free' (Wilbush, 1982). Finally much of the content of cultural attitudes to, and behaviour during the climacteric, may be peculiar to a particular cultural group and defy generalisation.

7

Methodological Issues in Climacteric Research

The preceding four chapters have been given over to an account of the empirical research which has been carried out on the symptomatology, psychosocial and sociocultural aspects of the climacteric in the general population of women. From time to time in the course of this account, attention has been drawn in individual studies, to certain inadequacies of the research design. This has been done with the intention of indicating that the conclusions reached by the authors of such studies, must be regarded with some reservations. This chapter is devoted to a fuller discussion of methodological issues, some of which are, and some of which are not, peculiar to climacteric research. We shall begin with a number of general points regarding research design before moving on to discuss two specific problems of method, both of which are central to climacteric research. These are, firstly, the operational methods that have been used to determine menopausal and climacteric status, and secondly the procedures used to assess climacteric symptomatology. We begin, however, with a discussion of some general design problems.

7.1. GENERAL CONSIDERATIONS

Perhaps the most frequent criticisms made of research design in preceding chapters has been of the unrepresentative nature of many of the 'general population' samples employed in studies. Frequently it is clear that the particular sample of women, although from the general population is, because of the authors sampling procedure, a biased one, usually in the direction of over representing upper socioeconomic groups. This means that, regardless of results and the adequacy of other aspects of the design, limitations are imposed on any extrapolation from such studies to women in general, particularly as it has been clearly established that social class has such a critical influence on women's responses during the climacteric (section 5.3).

The reason why samples tend to be unrepresentative lies in the variety of sources from which women have been obtained. Some researchers have used volunteers, obtained either through personal contact or by advertising, which explains perhaps why so many of the women come from higher social class groups. Others have selected patients from general practice lists which, depending on the location and type of the practice, may or may not produce a representative sample. Still others have relied on clinical populations. Indeed, only in a minority of the studies reviewed in Chapters 3, 4, 5 and 6 have subjects been selected by proper random sampling procedures.

An equally serious problem in climacteric research is the lack of consistency between studies in many aspects of research design. A brief inspection of Tables 2.1, 3.1, 5.1 and 6.1 will suffice to demonstrate this point. These variations have already been commented on in the relevant chapters, but let us consider two of these inconsistencies in a little more detail, namely, those of sample size and measuring instruments.

In the surveys of symptom prevalence among the general population of climacteric women reviewed in Chapter 3 (see Table 3.1) the size of the samples varied considerably from some 150 in the survey by Kaufert and Syrotuik (1981) to almost 3000 in that by Jaszmann et al. (1969b). Sample size per se is not as critical an issue as is sometimes thought (see Hamilton, 1974, Chapter 7). What is more important is that the sample be a genuinely random one. A small random sample, even of 150, is without doubt superior to a large biased one of 3000. Although in the examples given above the reverse is the case, as in fact the smaller sample is biased and the large one random. A large biased sample, however, merely increases systematic error and confounds the problems arising from its unrepresentativeness, especially if the object is to obtain an estimate of general population parameters. Assuming that it is randomly selected, the larger a sample the greater is the reduction of chance error. However, should a sample be extremely large, then differences between groups of subjects may achieve statistical significance, although these differences may be of very small *absolute* magnitude. Thus statistically significant findings may emerge with large samples which are in fact, for all practical purposes, worthless.

Probably a more critical variation between studies relates to assessment procedures. The procedures by which both independent and dependent variables are measured are often ad hoc, and peculiar to that particular study. This renders any direct comparison of studies researching the same area difficult, if similar parameters are being assessed by quite different measuring instruments.

There is in fact no shortage of well designed and standardised tests and scales to assess various psychological and social characteristics, and indeed some researchers in this field have availed themselves of such methods. Uphold and Susman (1981), for example, used the Dyadic Adjustment Scale developed by Spanier (1976) to assess marital adjustment, in contrast with the series of ad hoc questions made up by Crawford and Hooper (1973) to assess the same variable. Similarly, despite the existence of the well designed and factorially valid Attitudes-Toward-Menopause Checklist developed by Neugarten et al. (1963), Maoz et al. (1970), in their later study of attitudes among Israeli women, made up their own measure using their less satisfactory gain-loss criteria. This method inevitably resulted in spurious relationships being found between women's attitudes and some of those aetiological factors thought to predispose women to develop different attitudes to the menopause, as similar criteria were used for both. This arose for example, when concern over loss of fertility was used as a criterion of a negative attitude, when one of the putative psychosexual factors determining this attitude was a desire to have more children (see section 6.1).

A not dissimilar situation arises with regard to menopausal status when it is self defined and used as an aetiological factor in relation to self reported symptoms. Again there is a confounding of the procedures by which the causal and outcome variables are measured. This brings us to two methodological problems which, unlike those just discussed, are problems peculiar to climacteric research. These are firstly, the problems of operationally defining menopausal and climacteric status, and secondly, the problem of satisfactorily and adequately measuring the most widely used dependent variable, namely, symptomatology.

7.2. OPERATIONAL DEFINITIONS OF MENOPAUSAL AND CLIMACTERIC STATUS

Conceptual definitions of menopause and climacteric have been provided at the very beginning of this volume in section 1.3. In doing so, the author closely followed those proposed by Utian and Serr (1976) and which are now generally accepted by climacteric researchers. (See editorial note in *Maturitas* by van Keep, 1979.) Operational definitions refer to the objective criteria by which a variable is actually measured. This is usually set out by the researcher in his description of the research design. That is, it is the precise operation by which the variable is to be measured. There is less consensus about these in respect to both menopausal and climacteric status.

Menopausal Status

In the majority of studies reviewed in this volume menopausal status has been defined in terms of changes in the menstrual pattern. In a few cases the unsatisfactory method of having women classify themselves as menopausal or not, has been used, e.g. Neugarten and Kraines (1965) and Crawford and Hooper (1973). As has been pointed out previously, this is unsatisfactory because of the possibility of confounding menopausal status and symptoms. That is, a woman who is experiencing certain symptoms in middle life may regard herself as menopausal for that very reason and vice versa. Indeed, the same bias may exist even if the women is so classified by a clinician or researcher on the basis of symptoms. The only satisfactory method so far developed, is to define menopausal status in relation to changes in the menstrual cycle.

Two different methods have been commonly used, that of McKinlay et al. (1972), which has tended to be used in UK studies, and that of

Jaszmann et al. (1969b) which has been used mainly in European studies. The two methods are compared in Table 7.1. As can be seen, in McKinlay's method pre and perimenopause are defined in terms of when the last menstrual cycle occurred. Using Jaszmann's method, this classification is based on changes in the pattern of the menstrual cycle. In both methods the postmenopause is defined in the same way. These two methods would naturally lead to some differences in classifying women as

Table 7.1

Comparison of two Methods of Defining Menopausal Status

Menopausal Status	McKinlay's Method	Jaszmann's Method
Premenopause	Menstruated within the last 3 months	Normal menses during preceding year.
Perimenopause	Last menstruated between 3 and 12 months ago	Menstrual pattern different i.e., more or fewer cycles than previously during preceding year.
Postmenopause	Did not menstruate within last 12 months	Did not menstruate in preceding year.

pre or perimenopausal. In the McKinlay method, if a woman experiences one cycle within the previous three months she is classed as premenopausal, even if there had been some irregularity during the nine months before. Such women would be classified by Jaszmann's method as perimenopausal. The result of these differences might be for the McKinlay method to misclassify a number of women as premenopausal who were really perimenopausal. This would be the case, for example, if a woman fortuitously menstruated within the previous three months, following a long period of missed cycles.

The advantages of using McKinlay's method on the other hand is that it is a more objective one, and only requires women to recall when their last period occurred. This can be quite accurate so long as the time interval is not in excess of about three years as there is a tendency, if it is longer than this for women to 'round off' to the nearest 5 or 10 years (McKinlay et al., 1972). Jaszmann's method requires a woman to make a judgement as to any change in menstrual pattern over the preceding year, in comparison with the year before. This is a more subjective criterion and is dependent on more detailed recall on the part of the woman. Both methods therefore, have their advantages and disadvantages, but for the purpose of empirical research a method based in some way on the menstrual cycle is clearly superior to one derived from self definition or reported symptoms, especially if the latter is also a dependent variable.

Climacteric Status

Another variation in method has been the age range from within which women have been sampled. The common research strategy has been to select women from within a predetermined age range, and categorise them as pre, peri or postmenopausal. As the majority of women experience the menopause within 45 to 50 years, it is customary to choose an age range so many years on either side of this period. This is done in order not to omit too many women having an early or a late menopause, and to adequately cover the climacteric period. The aim, that is, is to have a group well representative of climacteric women.

The age ranges commonly used have been 45 to 54, 40 to 55 and 40 to 60 years. However, because of the difficulty of determining when the climacteric, when defined as the transition from being reproductive to non-reproductive, begins, any age limit is essentially an arbitrary one. Nevertheless, some sort of consensus on this point is desirable in order to allow comparability of studies. Certainly if the mean age of the menopause is somewhere around 50 years and if ovarian dysfunction, as stated earlier, may begin some ten years before that event and continue some years thereafter (see section 1.1), then the narrower age range of 45 to 54 years would seem inadequate. A wider one would seem more appropriate.

A few researchers have also included pre and postclimacteric women in their studies. While this is not absolutely necessary, it is of added interest as it allows age trends to be observed, sometimes, as has been seen, highly revealingly. See, for example, the surveys by Neugarten and Kraines (1965), van Keep and Kellerhals (1975), Wood (1979), Bungay et al. (1980) and Greene and Cooke (1980), all reviewed in section 3.2.

7.3. THE ASSESSMENT OF CLIMACTERIC SYMPTOMS

Symptoms are the most commonly used measure of women's reactions at the climacteric, and as we have seen the most widespread method of assessing them has been by means of a checklist. That is, a list of symptoms are drawn up and women are asked to check which symptoms they are currently experiencing, usually on a present-absent basis. A typical checklist of this sort was illustrated in Table 1.2. Items for these checklists have generally been selected on the basis of a review of the literature or because, in the author's view, they are 'typical or common menopausal symptoms'. As has been pointed out at the beginning of this volume (section 1.2) the use of the term 'menopausal symptoms' is an unfortunate one, as it seems to imply that the event of the menopause bears some *causal* relationship to these symptoms. As we have seen in this volume, these symptoms have many origins. The present author favours the more generic term climacteric symptoms, if climacteric is used in a wide sense to refer to that phase in the ageing process during which a women passes from a reproductive to a non-reproductive state. This implies that climacteric symptoms are many and may have many origins (section 1.3).

Before proceeding to discuss the methodology of assessing climacteric symptoms, it is first necessary to dispose of a common but misdirected criticism of such attempts. This position is well represented in the quote below from Davis (1983), who highlights two 'insoluble difficulties' in assessing climacteric symptoms:

> (1) symptoms, being predominately psychological in nature, are almost impossible to define objectively and consistently across different groups, nor can the severity of such symptoms be objectively measured; (2) regardless of the refinement of various instruments for collecting information, heavy reliance must be placed on material reported by the respondents themselves (p.179).

The following response can be made to these arguments. Symptoms by definition, are subjective phenomenon, and who but the person experiencing them is in the best position to report them. They are often the first indications of illness and medical practice, therefore, relies heavily on these subjective experiences. The object of any assessment instrument is merely to order these subjective experiences and reports, not to arrive at some definitive 'objective' measure of them. The history of clinical psychometry demonstrates convincingly that this can be done in a reliable and valid way (Anastasi, 1976). Finally, inconsistencies across different groups need not reflect on the measuring instrument, but may reflect differences between populations.

Climacteric Symptom Checklists

The checklist method of eliciting symptoms has been criticised, in the climacteric literature, on the grounds that providing a list of symptoms for subjects to check off is likely to lead to a reporting of more symptoms than would be the case if women were asked spontaneously to report their symptoms, especially if the subject is aware that the investigation is to do with the menopause (McKinlay and Jefferys, 1974). This, indeed, was observed to be the case by Thompson et al. (1973), who found that an open ended questionnaire produced fewer symptoms than did a checklist. Van Keep (1975), while confirming this, noted that while many women reported vasomotor symptoms spontaneously, fewer spontaneously reported other somatic and psychological symptoms. It will be recalled that Wright (1980) obtained similar results with Navajo women, as did Davis (1983) with Newfoundland women (section 6.2). It is a moot point however as to whether the checklist method leads to more over reporting of symptoms than the open ended method does to the under reporting of symptoms.

In fact, it is well known that in clinical practice in general, patients report few symptoms spontaneously and that it is part of a clinician's skill to elicit other relevant symptoms by careful and systematic probing, in order to arrive at a correct diagnosis. The tendency for individuals to report fewer symptoms spontaneously than they would in response to specific questioning, is therefore a widespread phenomenon and not one that is confined to the climacteric, nor as some have suggested (Wilbush, 1982) to non-Western communities. Indeed, because of this Wright advises that 'researchers in all cultures should ask explicitly if a respondent has experienced specific symptoms, rather than asking generally if there have been any health problems or bodily changes since the ending of periods' (p.61). This would appear to be sound advice, since in balancing the risks of over reporting against that of under reporting symptoms, the former is probably to be preferred.

In effect, almost all researchers have favoured providing a list of symptoms as being the most practical of the two approaches. In addition, the checklist method, or similar techniques, are the most commonly used ones in medical, psychiatric, epidemiological and clinical psychological research. This is because it allows a greater measure of control over subjects' responses and is therefore scientifically more acceptable, especially from the point of replication, than is the open ended method. While the foregoing are conceptual points, criticisms can be made of the way in which checklists have been used in climacteric research. As has been noted previously, checklists assembled in this way have been of varying lengths, symptoms are generally rated in terms of the symptoms' presence or absence and the results have been reported in varying ways. Each of these points will now be elaborated in turn.

Length of Checklists

How many and which symptoms will be included in a checklist will obviously reflect the researcher's view as to the nature and diversity of climacteric symptomatology. As the climacteric occurs over a lengthy period of time, affects most of the body's system and has many origins — physiological, social and psychological — symptoms could de facto be assumed to be unlimited. In practice the length of checklists reflects the comprehensiveness of the study, and the resources available to the research group, as much as views as to what constitutes the climacteric syndrome. There does, however, seem to be some consensus about a core group of symptoms, as some symptoms repeatedly appear in most checklists (see for example, Table 3.6). Nevertheless, some sort of consistency regarding which symptoms, and how many should be included, would be desirable from the point of view of comparing and replicating studies. In section 7.4 of this Chapter a more rational and empirical method for selecting symptoms, than has been used hitherto, will be outlined.

Rating of Symptoms

Simply rating a symptom as present or absent, as is often the practice in climacteric research, is generally unsatisfactory since such a measure tends to be less sensitive than one in which the symptom is rated in terms of severity. This is particularly important in regard to symptoms at the climacteric which, by and large, are non-specific and can occur at any age and in many other groups of subjects and conditions. Such insensitivity is likely to obscure differences between groups which may emerge more clearly when symptoms are rated according to severity. Many people will admit, for example, to 'feeling depressed over the past month or so'. What is important is just how depressed they have felt. This insensitivity could also account for the high prevalance rates of symptoms reported in some of the surveys reviewed in Chapter 3. Some sort of assessment, therefore, of the severity or frequency of occurrence of a symptom is necessary, in order to arrive at a more sensitive measure of the *degree* of distress being experienced by individual climacteric women or by particular subgroups of women.

Reporting Checklist Results

In reporting the responses of women to checklists, symptoms have either been dealt with singly, in which case the percentage of women complaining of each symptom is given, or else symptoms are summated to yield a total symptom score for each woman. In some instances symptoms are grouped into subcategories, for example, physical, psychosomatic and psychological, as in the survey by Neugarten and Kraines (1965), or as in that by Severne (1979), into Circulatory and Nervosity Indices.

The criticisms made above regarding the insensitivity of rating symptoms as present or absent applies equally well to reporting symptoms singly, since an important consideration in assessing an individual woman's distress is not just the presence of an individual symptom, but also the number of other symptoms she is experiencing. However summating symptoms is also generally unsatisfactory since by grouping diverse symptoms together, variation in different *types* of symptoms are obscured. This was seen early on in the review of symptom surveys in Chapter 3, where, in the survey by Jaszmann et al. (1969b), the breakdown of symptoms into subgroups, revealed differing temporal relationships to menopausal status which were obscured when a total symptom count was used (see Figure 3.1). The most obvious example of this occurs when vasomotor symptoms, which are known to be the symptoms most associated with oestrogen deficiency and which behave in a characteristic way in relation to the menopause, are included in total symptom counts. This was most clearly seen when the results of the two IHF surveys were compared (see Figures 3.4 and 3.5). Furthermore, as we have seen in Chapters 5 and 6, and shall see again in Chapter 8, different causal factors exercise their effect on different types of symptoms. Unfortunately, when researchers have subdivided non-vasomotor symptoms into subgroups, this has often been done in an arbitrary way.

In general, therefore, researchers in the past have tended to assess climacteric symptoms by means of unsophisticated ad hoc measures and with few exceptions have made no attempt to develop composite *scales* with satisfactory psychometric properties. The one exception to the ad hoc trend over the years has been the Blatt Menopausal Index, which has been used in a number of studies. This scale, first described in the early fifties (Blatt et al., 1953) is identical to the Kupperman Index (Kupperman et al., 1953) by which name it is also known (see section 2.3). Although the eleven symptoms on this scale are rated in terms of severity and weighted according to their importance, the weighting system is a completely arbitrary one. In addition, this scale yields a total score in which there is a confounding of vasomotor with other symptoms, and since the former receive the highest weighting, this index is primarily a measure of vasomotor symptoms.

There is therefore a need for a satisfactory, agreed-on instrument for assessing symptomatology at the climacteric. Since there is undoubted agreement that the symptoms women may experience during the climacteric are diverse and many, a first step in the proper appraisal and assessment of these symptoms, is the clarification of the relationship *among* symptoms and the identification of subcategories of symptoms using *empirical* methods, as opposed to previous arbitrary methods. An empirical technique for doing this is factor analysis. This method has proved to be of value in analysing symptoms in other multi-symptom conditions, notably in psychiatric depression (Eysenck, 1970), where differing interpretations of that syndrome have existed. Furthermore, as a first step in the construction of a proper assessment procedure, a study of the factorial composition of a symptom complex is essential (Eysenck, 1953; Lawley and Maxwell, 1963). To date four such studies of climacteric symptoms have been carried out.

7.4. FACTOR ANALYTIC STUDIES OF CLIMACTERIC SYMPTOMS

Factor analysis is a well established statistical method for initially exploring symptoms complexes. This technique entails analysing the relationship among various symptoms, for the purpose of determining which symptoms cluster together to form subgroups, each possibly having a different aetiology. If, for example, the view of those writers who claim that most symptoms at the climacteric are associated with oestrogen deficiency is correct (section 2.1), then one would expect symptoms to form a single cluster or factor, having a single aetiology. If, however, there are a number of different aetiological variables operating on climacteric symptoms, then it would be anticipated that a number of different factors would emerge, reflecting different clusters of symptoms, each possibly with a different aetiology. So far four factor analytic studies of climacteric symptoms have been reported. The first such study was carried out by the present author (Greene, 1976) among a clinical population of women. This study was subsequently replicated in a similar group of Indian women by Indira and Murthy (1980b). This was followed by two not dissimilar studies, one in Canada by Kaufert and Syrotuik (1981), the other in Norway by Mikkelsen and Holte (1982), using general population samples. These studies will now be discussed.

Greene (1976)

This study was carried out by the present author, firstly for the purpose of investigating the inter-relationships between symptoms presented by women at the climacteric, and secondly for the purpose of producing, if possible, a more rational and empirically based method of assessing symptoms at the climacteric. A checklist of symptoms was administered to a group of climacteric women and the data submitted to a principal factor analysis.

Subjects consisted of 50 middle aged women successively referred to a Hormone Replacement Therapy Clinic in the city of Glasgow, Scotland, by their general practitioners. All women, age range 40 to 55 years, had initially gone to their general practitioners complaining of vasomotor symptoms together with, in varying degrees, a number of other somatic and psychological symptoms. All women were seen by a consultant gynaecologist who confirmed clinically that they were climacteric. The criteria for this was that they were experiencing vasomotor symptoms of natural onset and that their periods had either stopped spontaneously within the past three years, or were currently irregular. Nineteen women had menstruated within the previous three months but had experienced some change in regularity and/or volume in the previous year (transitional menopause); 13 had last menstruated betweeen 3 and 12 months previously (perimenopausal) and 18 between 1 and 3 years ago (postmenopausal). Mean age of the group was 49.3 years. Before beginning hormone therapy each women completed a number of psychological tests including a 45 item self administered symptom checklist. The symptoms were derived from a search of the literature and included all symptoms traditionally thought to be associated with the climacteric. The format of the checklist was based on that of the widely used Symptom Rating Test of Kellner and Sheffield (1973). Items were worded to facilitate understanding and subjects were required to rate the extent to which they were bothered by each symptom on a 4-point severity rating — not at all; a little; quite a bit; extremely.

Before carrying out the factor analysis, items which proved to be ambiguous and those of low frequency (less than 5 per cent) were discarded. The remaining items, of which there were 30, were scored 0 to 3 according to their severity, and intercorrelated, using product-moment coefficients. The resulting matrix was then sumbmitted to a principal factor analysis. Significant factors, as determined by the Cattell scree test (Cattell, 1966) were rotated to oblique simple structure by the direct oblimin method. Three factors, accounting for in all 38 per cent of the variance, emerged as significant. Table 7.2 shows rotated factor loadings. The size of the factor loading is a measure of the degree to which each symptom correlates with each factor and therefore reflects the relative importance of each symptom to each factor.

Symptoms are listed in Table 7.2 according to the size of their factor loadings on each factor. As can be seen Factor I, which has high loadings on symptoms 1 to 14, is readily identifiable as a psychological factor, as opposed to Factor II (symptoms 15 to 22), which appears to be a general somatic factor. Factor III has specific loadings on only three symptoms, and is clearly identifiable as a vasomotor factor. The remaining five symptoms show no specific loading on any one factor. Table 7.2 also shows correlation between each of the factors. All correlations are low and insignificant, indicating virtually independent relationships between each of the factors. The factor structure emerging is therefore that of three identifiable and independent factors or clusters of symptoms.

What this means is that the non-vasomotor symptoms presented by this group of climacteric women fall into two major clusters. One of these consists of psychological, the other somatic symptoms, neither group being associated with each other, *nor* with the smaller cluster of vasomotor symptoms. Hot flushes in fact emerged quite independently from these two groups, being associated, in terms of factor loadings, with no psychological and only two somatic symptoms. These were 'cold hands and feet', which could be regarded as a vasomotor symptom, and 'aches in back of neck and skull'. Once again therefore vasomotor symptoms are seen to behave quite differently from other symptoms. Were, for example, the unitary view of symptoms to be a valid interpretation of climacteric symptoms, then only a single significant factor or cluster, with positive loadings on most items, would have emerged. The type of factor structure obtained suggests tentatively that a different causal mechanism may be operating in each case, and naturally raises further doubt as to the oestrogenic basis of the accompanying psychological and somatic symptoms.

Table 7.2

Rotated Factor Loadings of Climacteric Symptoms

	Symptoms	Factors I	II	III
1.	Feeling unhappy or depressed.	78	08	12
2.	Feeling tense or wound up.	76	-34	05
3.	Crying spells.	76	04	-15
4.	Feeling tired or lacking in energy.	71	16	-27
5.	Lost interest in most things.	68	03	-09
6.	Attacks of panic.	63	11	-05
7.	Worrying needlessly.	57	-45	23
8.	Heart pounding quickly or strongly.	48	23	-12
9.	Muscle pains, aches or rheumatism.	47	03	32
10.	Excitable.	44	03	26
11.	Sleep disturbed.	44	15	25
12.	Poor concentration.	42	26	25
13.	Irritable.	40	31	05
14.	Restless or jumpy.	38	28	29
15.	Blind spots before eyes.	-06	57	-10
16.	Crawling feelings over skin.	36	57	-09
17.	Parts of body feel numb or tingling.	11	52	17
18.	Feelings of suffocation.	-05	52	00
19.	Headaches.	-29	49	24
20.	Pressure or tightness in head or body.	14	47	29
21.	Weight gain.	20	47	-21
22.	Feeling dizzy or faint.	29	46	01
23.	Aches in back of neck and skull.	16	05	69
24.	Hot flushes.	01	-24	61
25.	Cold hands and feet.	09	04	49
26.	Heavy periods.	-31	39	43
27.	Poor memory.	34	14	41
28.	Poor appetite.	28	-05	03
29.	Breast pains.	16	16	-20
30.	Constipation or diarrhoea.	-31	39	43

Decimal points omitted
Factor intercorrelations: I v II = 0.21; I v III = 0.10; II v III = 0.04

From Greene (1976)

Indira and Murthy (1980b)

The foregoing factor analytic study was subsequently replicated by Indira and Murthy (1980b) among a population of Indian women. This consisted of 105 women in the age range 36 to 50 years, all of whom were attending a gynaecological outpatient clinic. Most of these women were either seeking help for a minor gynaecological problem or were attending for a routine check-up. Symptoms were assessed by means of the same 30 symptom checklist used by Greene (1976), each symptom being similarly rated in severity. The resulting correlation matrix was then submitted to a principal components analysis, which was then rotated by the varimax method.

The first three factors resulting from rotation accounted for some 68 per cent of the variance. As in the study by Greene (1976), these three factors were easily identified as a psychological, a somatic and a vasomotor one. In regard to the actual symptoms making up these factors, there was close agreement between the two studies on the psychological symptoms. For the vasomotor factor, hot flushes and sweating had again by far the highest factor loadings, and again this factor stood out as independent from the other two. There was less agreement between the two studies about the individual symptoms making up the somatic factor, a difference that Indira and Murthy attribute to cultural variation in the experiencing and reporting of physical symptoms.

The importance of this factorial study is that in respect both to method and findings, it is an exact replication of a previous study. Furthermore, it has shown that symptoms among a population of climacteric women in India, form a factor structure *identical* to that of a similar group of women from an entirely different cultural setting, although there is some difference in the individual symptoms contributing to each factor. This is a good example of crosscultural continuity in structure with variation in content.

Kaufert and Syrotuik (1981)

This third factor analysis of climacteric symptoms differs from the two previous ones in that the study sample was a general population one. It has earlier been referred to in section 3.2 where the relationship between the symptom factors and menopausal status was discussed. It will be recalled that symptoms were assessed by means of two scales, one measuring vasomotor the other psychological symptoms. These scales had been derived from a factor analysis of a checklist of eleven menopausal symptoms taken from the Climacteric Index used in the IHF surveys, together with seven 'filler' symptoms. Of these eighteen symptoms, eleven are the same as, or have their equivalent in the list used by Greene (1976) and Indira and Murthy (1980b).

The response of the 148 women to each of the symptoms was then factor analysed using the principal component method. It was found that four factors yielded the most meaningfull solution. These were then rotated using the oblique method. The resulting factor structure is shown in Table 7.3. The first of these factors yielded highest loadings on the

Table 7.3

Rotated Factor Loadings of Climacteric Symptoms

Symptoms	I	II	III	IV
1. Irritability.	64	10	-23	-09
2. Tiredness.	56	-04	-09	-03
3. Depression.	50	-21	43	04
4. Nervous tension.	49	-02	04	00
5. Trouble sleeping.	45	02	04	-13
6. Diarrhoea	04	57	-02	02
7. Upset stomach.	-16	56	14	-09
8. Headaches.	34	37	01	03
9. Short of breath.	24	36	-03	06
10. Dizziness	07	29	15	-17
11. Aches and pains in joints.	-10	05	47	-18
12. Pins and needles.	00	-01	48	02
13. Backaches.	13	07	39	05
14. Sore throat	00	01	48	02
15. Hot flushes.	03	-12	03	65
16. Night sweats	03	05	01	64
17. Cough.	19	18	06	35
18. Rapid heart beat.	15	02	12	01

Decimal points omitted

Adapted from Kaufert and Syrotuik (1981)

symptoms of tiredness, irritability, depression, nervous tension and trouble sleeping and was accordingly labelled a psychological factor. The second and third factors, for reasons that are not entirely clear, the authors dismiss as 'without relevance in this discussion'. Nevertheless, both these factors have their highest loadings exclusively on somatic symptoms — numbers 6 to 14. The fourth factor had high loadings only on the symptoms of hot flushes and night sweats, and was clearly a vasomotor factor.

In general terms therefore, the factor *structure* emerging in this study, although carried out on quite a different type of population, bears a close resemblance to that obtained by both Greene (1976) and Indira and Murthy (1980b). First of all, three *types* of clusters of symptoms emerge, and while Kaufert and Syrotuik obtained two somatic factors this could be due either to their method of factor analysis or to the inclusion of filler items, all of which were somatic. Secondly, although there is some variation between the studies with regard to the absolute magnitude of factor loadings, in regard to relative loadings, there is almost perfect agreement. That is, of the eleven symptoms having an equivalent in the list used by Greene (1976), the six symptoms which had their highest loadings on the psychological factor, and the five symptoms with their highest loadings on the somatic factors in the Kaufert and Syrotuik study, also had their highest loadings on the same factors in Greene's study. Thirdly, and perhaps more importantly, is the common finding that vasomotor symptoms form a separate group quite independent from all other symptoms.

Mikkelsen and Holte (1982)

In this final factor analytic study, aspects of which relating symptoms to menopausal status were also reported in section 3.2, the study sample was also taken from the general population. It will be recalled that climacteric symptoms had been measured by means of six scales derived from a factor analysis of a 21 symptom checklist. To arrive at these scales, the symptoms of the 139 women were rated on a 3-point rating scale of severity and their intercorrelations submitted to a principal factor analysis. Using a varimax rotation six factors were extracted. One of these factors obtained high loadings only on the symptoms of hot flushes, excessive sweating and vaginal dryness and was accordingly labelled a vasomotor factor. Two psychological factors, termed 'mood lability' and 'nervousness', emerged. The other three factors consisted of a general somatic factor with high loadings on seven symptoms, and two highly specific factors, one containing 'urinary' symptoms the other only one symptom — 'shortness of breath'. Symptoms associated with each factor are shown in Table 7.4 together with their factor loadings.

The outcome of this factor analytic study of climacteric symptoms concurs with all previous ones in finding, firstly that vasomotor symptoms form a group independently from all other symptoms, and secondly that these other symptoms in turn form separate groups, which can be identified as psychological and somatic factors. Certainly, this

Table 7.4

Symptoms with High Loadings on each Factor

Symptoms According to Category	Factor Loadings
Vasomotor	
excessive sweating	77
hot flushes	68
vaginal dryness	36
Mood liability	
moodiness	83
irritability	78
feeling depressed	60
Nervousness	
other sleep problems	63
nervousness	59
difficulties in falling asleep	46
palpitations	36
General somatic	
muscle and joint pains	68
numbness and stiffness	58
fatigue	51
loss of feeling in hands and feet	50
back pains	50
dizziness	46
headaches	35
Urinary problems	
frequent urination	70
involuntary urination	55
Shortness of breath	
shortness of breath	52

Adapted from Mikkelsen and Holte (1982)

present study produced two of the former and three of the latter, but in general terms the *type* of factor structure is the same.

Discussion of Factor Analytic Studies

Thus, all four of these factorial studies of the symptoms presented by women during the climacteric, have produced an essentially similar *type* of factor structure, regardless of whether the study sample is a clinical or general population one. In this regard both Kaufert and Syrotuik (1981) and Mikkelsen and Holte (1982) have criticised Greene (1976) on the grounds that that study was carried out on a clinical population. However since factor analysis is based on the intercorrelations *between* symptoms there seems to be no a priori reason why the factorial structure obtained from a clinical population should, in any substantial way, be different from that derived from a general population. And indeed, as has been seen, there is no substantial difference between any of these studies and the essential *nature* of the factor structure.

Certainly both the factor analyses carried out on general population samples produced more factors than did those carried out on clinical populations, but this has probably nothing to do with the nature of the sample. How many factors should be extracted from a factor analysis is a moot point, and different factorial procedures may give different numbers. Differences in the number of factors produced is therefore more likely to be a function of the particular statistical method adopted. Had either Kaufert and Syrotuik (1981) and Mikkelsen and Holte (1982) *imposed* a three factor solution, the resulting factor structure would probably have been the same as those of Greene (1976) and Indira and Murthy (1980b). In this context the extraction of four factors on the basis of 18 symptoms by Kaufert and Syrotuik (1981), and of as many as six, by Mikkelsen and Holte (1982), from only 21 symptoms is somewhat unusual. Factor analysis is essentially a reductionist procedure, having the object of accounting for a wide range of items by as few variables as possible. Furthermore, no statistical test seems to have been used in either study to determine the significance of factors. Indeed, a factor based on one symptom, as was the 'shortness of breath' factor in the Mikkelsen and Holte (1982) study, can scarcely, by definition, be regarded as a factor at all. Thus, a three factor solution can be considered to be the most parsimonious and valid type of structure.

The finding that non-vasomotor climacteric symptoms fall into two main clusters, one psychological the other physical, is not, in fact, an unusual one. Hamilton (1959; 1960), for example, in factor analyses of his widely used Anxiety and Depression Rating Scales, both of which have been used in climacteric research (see especially section 2.3), found that for both these scales, factors corresponding to somatic and psychological symptoms emerged. From a practical consideration, the rationale for categorising non-specific symptoms reported by women at the climacteric into two major groups, psychological and somatic, and treating these separately from each other, and also separately from vasomotor symptoms, would appear to be a sound one.

A Climacteric Symptom Rating Scale

It is clear, therefore, that in assessing symptoms of women during the climacteric, it is important that the three main categories of symptoms should be measured separately. Factor analytic studies can also provide an empirical and rational method for constructing such measuring instruments. On the basis of the factorial study carried out by the present author, two scales were constructed to measure non-vasomotor symptoms — one to measure psychological, the other somatic symptoms.

For this purpose items with factor loadings greater than 0.40 on one factor and less than 0.30 on the other were selected. This was done to maintain the independence of the final two scales. This gave in all 18 items, 11 psychological and 7 somatic. These symptoms were then weighted according to their factor loading. Those with a factor loading greater than 0.50 were given a weighting of 2, and those with a loading less than 0.50 were given a weighting of 1. The final format of the scale is shown in Table 7.5. For scoring purposes, the scores of a subject on each item, using the original 0-3 severity rating, are multiplied by their weight and are summated to give a total score for each subscale. Subsequently the reliability of both scales was tested using the test-retest method. Thirty climacteric women completed the scale again after an interval of one week and reliability coefficients calculated. For the Psychological Scale this came out at 0.89 and for the Somatic Scale at 0.85, both of which are acceptably high. The end result therefore, is two empirically constructed, factorially valid and reliable scales for measuring non-vasomotor climacteric symptoms. These formed the two scales used in the survey of symptoms among climacteric women previously discussed in section 3.2 (Greene and Cooke, 1980).

It should be noted that the actual symptoms included in these two scales correspond closely to the checklists used in the studies discussed in Chapters 2, 3, 4 and 5. However, as indicated above the implication of factor analysis is that each of these three categories of symptoms —

Table 7.5

A Climacteric Symptom Rating Scale

Please indicate the extent to which you are bothered at the moment by any of these symptoms by placing a tick in the appropriate box.

Symptoms	Not at all	A little	Quite a bit	Extremely
1. Feeling tired or lacking in energy.				
2. Feeling dizzy or faint.				
3. Heart beating quickly or strongly.				
4. Pressure or tightness in head or body.				
5. Feeling tense or wound up.				
6. Parts of body feel numb or tingling.				
7. Loss of interest in most things.				
8. Feeling unhappy or depressed.				
9. Headaches.				
10. Attacks of panic.				
11. Difficulty in concentrating.				
12. Weight gain.				
13. Difficulty in sleeping.				
14. Excitable.				
15. Blind spots before eyes.				
16. Crying spells.				
17. Feelings of suffocation.				
18. Worrying needlessly.				

Scoring:

Each item is given a 0—3 rating depending on its reported severity. These ratings are multiplied by a weight, as shown below, to yield a total score for both subscales.

Psychological Scale			Somatic Scale	
Items	Weight		Items	Weight
1, 5, 7, 8, 10, 18	2		6, 15, 17	2
3, 11, 13, 14, 16	1		2, 4, 9, 12	1

Vasomotor symptoms and symptoms of atrophic vaginitis may be incorporated into this format, or may be assessed some other way as required e.g. daily or weekly flush count.

vasomotor, somatic, psychological — may have a different aetiology, and that in research into the aetiology of climacteric symptoms it follows that each should be treated separately. Certainly, it has been amply demonstrated in other parts of this volume that vasomotor symptoms behave quite differently from all other symptoms. As we shall see in the next chapter, there are also good reasons for believing that somatic symptoms on the one hand, and psychological ones on the other, may also be influenced by different aetiological variables.

8

Life Events During the Climacteric

In the preceding chapter methodological issues in climacteric research have been discussed in some detail. In doing so a number of criticisms have been made of the overall quality of research in this area, and a number of suggestions have been put forward to improve its quality. Perhaps the central issue of this problem, as has already been pointed out, is the ad hoc nature of much of the research methods. This penultimate chapter is given over to an account of a piece of climacteric research carried out by the present author within the methodological framework of what is now a well established research area. The area is that of life event research, and the work to be described represents an attempt to examine psychosocial aspects of the climacteric, using the methodology of one of the mainstream areas of current social science and medical research. By doing this, the results of climacteric research can be better evaluated, by being seen in relation to research findings in other fields and thereby integrated into the existing body of knowledge. This then is the overall purpose of this chapter. We begin with an account of the methodology, which over the years has been developed in life event research, before going onto describe and discuss the research study itself.

8.1. LIFE EVENT RESEARCH

Life event research denotes that field of research which is concerned with the association between the onset of illness and the occurrence of recent events or changes in the individual's physical and social environment. The notion that the occurrence of discrete life events, particularly stressful ones, may precipitate physical, psychosomatic or psychiatric conditions is not a new one. Such ideas have a long history both in popular and scientific thinking. However, it was not until within the last decade and a half that the systematic study of stressful life events and their relation to illness was developed. In this relatively short period of time a vast research literature had appeared.

It is not the intention of this author to review this literature, as full and detailed accounts of the results emerging from life event research over these years are well documented in numerous other books (Dohrenwend and Dohrenwend, 1974; Gunderson and Rahe, 1974; Brown and Harris, 1978; Dohrenwend and Dohrenwend, 1981; Henderson et al., 1981). Rather, some of the ways in which life events have been elicited and measured will be considered in order to illustrate the conceptual and methodological basis of this approach. Among researchers into life events, the idea of stress has been conceptualised, and therefore measured, in different ways. The three most prominent methods are those of Holmes and Rahe (1967), Paykel et al. 1971) and Brown et al. (1973). A brief account of these three approaches now follows.

Holmes and Rahe's Method

It was the pioneering work of these authors in the mid-sixties in overcoming the previous inherent circularity of attempting to measure stress by its effects, that is, in terms of the illness or symptoms it was causing, that led to contemporary systematic research into life event stress as we now know it. Holmes and Rahe (1967) saw stress in terms of the amount of change or adjustment that an event would demand from an individual. Therefore, both pleasant and unpleasant experiences may be regarded as stressful, and require some degree of social readjustment. Readjustment is defined as the intensity and length of time necessary to accommodate an event, regardless of the desirability of the event.

Their original measure consisted of a checklist of 43 discrete events, the degree of change or adjustment necessitated by each being determined by a method of quantification based on consensus scaling. This was done by having a group of subjects assign to each event a rating, based on the amount of change in accustomed pattern of life that event would require from the average person, irrespective of its desirability. These ratings were expressed in relation to marriage, which was assigned a fixed score of 50. The result is a checklist of events, each given a weight derived from the means of these ratings. Subsequently, for any individual the weights of each event reported are summated to yield a Total Life Change Score, which is thus based on a population consensus, independent of the individual's own reaction to the event. The latter is usually the presence of illness or symptoms. This procedure, as has been said, overcomes the hitherto inherent circularity of attempting to measure stress by its effects. In most life event research, events experienced by the subject are recorded in retrospect from within a fixed time period, six months or one year, prior to the onset of the illness or symptoms.

Paykel's Method

In general principles the method of measuring life events developed by Eugene Paykel and his colleagues is similar to that of Holmes and Rahe. It too is a checklist approach in which the severity of the effect of an event is based on consensually derived judgements. However, there are some important differences. Paykel and his co-workers (Paykel et al., 1971) conceive of stress in terms of the degree of upset produced by the event, arguing that unpleasant events will have a different effect on individuals, even although they may require the same amount of readjustment according to Holmes and Rahe's criteria. This view has been supported by some research work which has shown that a measure based on the undesirability of an event is a better predictor of illness than life change scores (Paykel et al., 1975; Tennant and Andrews, 1978).

Paykel's method of arriving at weights for different life events also differs from that of Holmes and Rahe. In their consensus study, subjects were asked to judge how upsetting each event might be for the average person. Judgement was by means of a 0 (least upsetting) to 20 (most upsetting) equal interval rating procedure with no event fixed (Paykel et al., 1971). Weights derived in this way have been found to be remarkably consistent and stable across different social and national groups (Paykel et al., 1976).

Paykel and his colleagues (Paykel et al., 1969) have also devised a system of categorising life events. In this system events are subdivided in three ways — Area of Activity (e.g. health, family, employment, marital, legal), their Desirability or Undesirability, and as to whether they involve people coming into (Entrances) or leaving (Exits), the social field of the subject. Weighted stress scores for these different categories of life events can also be calculated as above. The end result is a 60 item event checklist which yields a Total Life Stress Score, based on these consensually derived weights, and separate life stress scores for different subcategories of life events. Although similar in principle, Paykel's method of measuring life events is a more refined one than that of Holmes and Rahe.

Brown's Method

Brown et al. (1973) departs from these other researchers in regarding the implications of an event for the *individual person* as the most critical factor, rather than any consensual rating of its importance. The logic of this is to produce a radically different way of eliciting events. In assessing the personal implication of the event for an individual, the context and circumstances surrounding the event must be taken into account. Accordingly, Brown and his colleagues dispense with the method of eliciting life events by means of the checklist approach, replacing this by a lengthy and extensive interview of the subject, carried out by specially trained interviewers. In this way details of all the circumstances surrounding any event and the context within which it occurs are obtained. It is on the basis of this information that the degree of 'contextual threat' of an event for the particular individual is arrived at by the research team, rather than by means of consensual weights. This approach is referred to as an investigator-based, as opposed to respondent-based method (Brown, 1981), in that it is left to the investigator, by use of systematic and skilled interviewing to collect sufficient information for a decision to be made as to whether a life event has occurred, and if so, the nature and severity of the threat involved. It is because of this that special training of the interviewers is required.

Brown's approach to assessing life events could be regarded as an over elaborate, judgemental and possibly a less replicable and objective procedure than those of others. Criticisms of this nature have been made of it by Shapiro (1979), who, in a lengthy critique of the methodology, concluded that 'the procedure seemed to be highly contaminated and guided by a philosophy that was largely subjectivist' (p.603). However, Parry et al. (1981), working in another research centre, have carried out an inter-rater agreement study of this method over a lengthy period of research. The reliability levels obtained led these authors to conclude that the Brown 'measure of threatening life events can be used reliably by research groups working independently' (p.134). Furthermore, as Andrews and Tennant (1978) have pointed out, despite these marked differences of method, the findings of Brown and Paykel and their respective colleagues are remarkably similar, especially regarding the influence of life events on psychiatric illness.

The outcome of 15 years of intensive research in this field has been that life event research has become both conceptually sophisticated and methodologically refined, with researchers developing increasingly more complex theoretical models to account for the relationship between life events and illness. No longer do researchers think in terms of this as a simple direct causal link, but a variety of other concepts have been introduced to explain the nature of this link. This has given rise to such concepts as vulnerability, moderating variables, symptom formation factors, long term difficulties, additivity and specificity of events and so on. These theoretical aspects of life event research will be further discussed in the final section of this chapter.

In the meantime, a piece of research carried out by the present author into the significance of life events during the climacteric will be described. In view of what has been said earlier regarding the climacteric being a time of psychosocial change for many women (section 5.1), the methodology developed within life event research would seem an appropriate and potentially fruitful framework within which to examine some other possible origins of the climacteric syndrome.

8.2. A STUDY OF LIFE EVENTS AND CLIMACTERIC SYMPTOMS

The conceptual and methodological framework that has been developed in the field of life event research has just been described. In this section the results of a study carried out by the present author within this framework, into the relationship between life events and symptoms among a sample of climacteric women living in the city of Glasgow, Scotland, will be described.

Methodology

Part of the methodology of this study has already been described in section 3.2 of this volume, where the association between different categories of symptoms and menopausal and climacteric status was reported. It will be recalled that for this sample of Scottish women only vasomotor symptoms showed any close temporal relationship to the time of the menopause. In contrast, the main increase in other symptoms occurred some time prior to the menopause in the early climacteric, and was only marginally associated with that event (see Figure 3.6). In this respect the findings of this survey were similar to those of others.

The main focus of this research, however, was on the relationship between life events and somatic and psychological symptoms reported by women during the climacteric, symptoms being assessed by means of the Climacteric Symptom Rating Scale described towards the end of section 7.4 (see Table 7.5). For the purposes of this study the climacteric was taken to be the age range 35 to 54 years, this particular age range being chosen on the basis of the definitions presented at the end of section 1.3. There, it was argued that if the climacteric is defined as the phase in the ageing process marking the transition from the reproductive to the non-reproductive stage of life, and that this is synonymous with ovarian failure, then such a process may begin some years before the menopause and continue for some years thereafter. In addition, as there is some variation in the age at menopause, a fairly wide age limit is necessary (see section 7.2). However, it must be kept in mind that exact age limits are purely arbitrary and serve only as working definitions. Within this age range menopausal status was determined by the method of McKinlay et al. (1972) as outlined in section 7.2.

In assessing life events the method devised by Paykel and his colleagues was followed (section 8.1). A non-directive semistructured interviewing technique was used to elicit those events which had been experienced by the subject in the previous twelve months, only those events rated as 'almost certainly independent' or 'probably independent' from symptoms being considered. These are events which, it is thought, are unlikely to have been a consequence of symptoms (Brown, 1972). A list of 63 events, most of which were taken from the existing life event literature was used. Each was clearly operationally defined beforehand. In scoring events the consensually derived weighting system devised by Paykey et al. (1976) was used. As indicated previously this method initially yields a Total Life Stress score for each individual, this being the sum of the weights of each life event experienced. Stress scores for different categories of life events were also calculated in this way.

Total Life Stress and Symptoms

Total Life Stress Scores (Paykel et al., 1976) were first calculated and examined in regard to climacteric and menopausal status (Greene and Cooke, 1980). This measure was found to be related to the former but not the latter. The relationship to the climacteric is illustrated in Figure 8.1 and shows that, like symptoms, Total Life Stress increases and peaks during the early part of this period. There was no tendency for women to experience more life events at the perimenopause than at any other time during the climacteric.

The question arising now is, to what extent is the concomitant increase in symptoms during the climacteric related to the increase in Total Life Stress? As it was still possible that some of the increase in symptoms was due to Total Life Stress and the menopause acting in conjuncton, a hierarchical stepwise multiple regression analysis was used to test these relationships. This allows one to determine not only the effect of each factor independently (that is Total Life Stress and menopausal status), but also any interactive effects of these factors working in conjunction can be seen. This method has been advocated by Cohen (1968) as an alternative to analysis of variance because of its flexibility. It can therefore be seen whether or not women are more liable to respond adversely to life stress during the perimenopause than at any other time. This can be done by calculating the significance of the Beta coefficients, which are standardised partial regression coefficients (Dartington, 1968).

These Beta coefficients can be seen in Table 8.1 together with their significance levels. As can be seen of the two independent factors, Total Life Stress shows the greater, and a significant, relationship to both symptom measures. There is a slight tendency for them to interact, especially on psychological symptoms but this effect is not significant. These results suggest therefore, that the increase in both somatic and psychological symptoms in climacteric women is, at least in part, a response to an increase in stress arising from life events. Being menopausal contributes little to this increase, nor does it act to any great extent to further enhance the effect of life events on symptoms. This group of women did not therefore appear to be more vulnerable to life stress at the time of the menopause.

So far it has been demonstrated that among this sample of urban Scottish women there is an increase in symptoms during the climacteric. There is also a simultaneous increase in the number of recent stressful life events at this time, the severity of which is directly associated with the

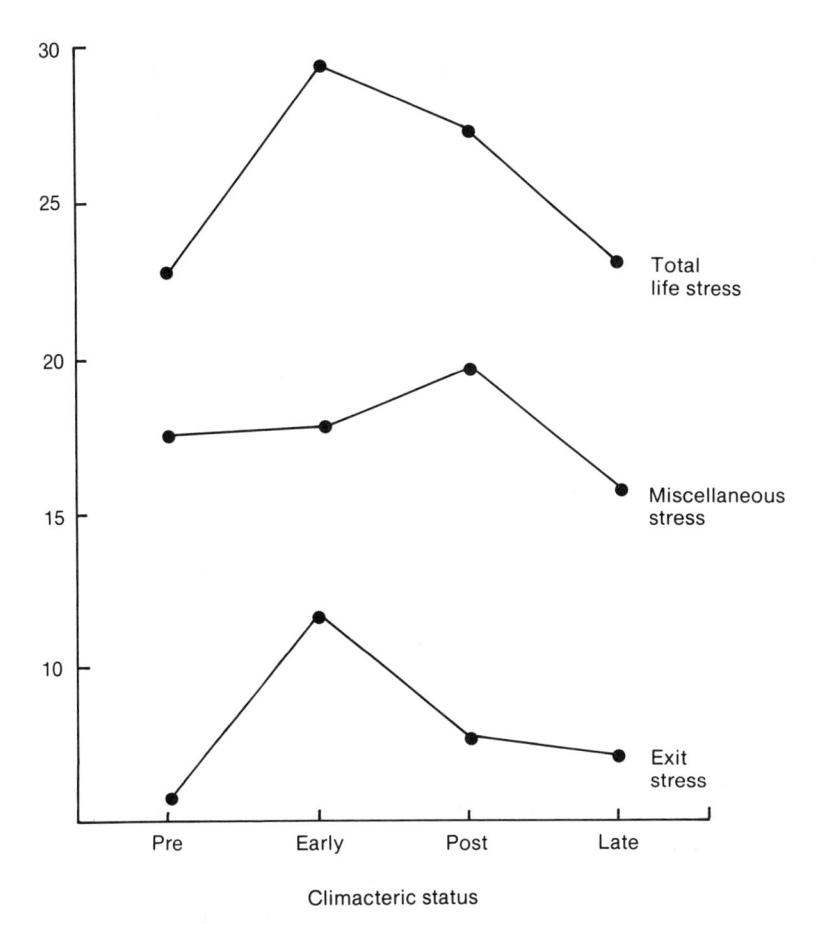

Figure 8.1 Mean scores for total life stress and its two main subcategories in relation to climacteric status. (from Greene, 1982)

severity of both psychological and somatic symptoms. It therefore seems reasonable to conclude at this stage that at least some of the increase in symptomatology during the climacteric is a response to a concomitant increase in stress at that time of life. This being so, in the context of the climacteric, an immediate question which comes to mind is whether this

Table 8.1

Significances of the Relationships between Total Life Stress, Menopausal Status and Symptoms

	Psychological Symptoms		Somatic Symptoms	
	Beta	F	Beta	F
Total life stress	2.04	5.39[a]	2.33	7.37[b]
Menopausal status	1.01	0.96	0.65	1.24
TLS × MS	1.20	0.79	0.76	0.33

a $P < 0.02$; b $P < 0.01$

Adapted from Greene and Cooke (1980)

increase in symptoms is a response to stressful life events in general, or whether particular types of life events are occurring, which are of special significance at that time of life. This of course takes us back to the notion of psychosocial transition previously discussed in section 5.1.

Types of Life Events

As the method of measuring life events was based on that of Paykel, this hypothesis was tested by first examining the types of life events women were being exposed to, using the categories devised by Paykel (Cooke and Greene, 1981). On the whole there was little difference between the area of activity categories or undesirability or otherwise of life events being experienced by women during the climacteric, and those reported by younger women (25 to 34 years) and older women (55 to 64 years). There was one marked exception to this. Exits, that is departures of others from the social field of the subject, were clearly more numerous among climacteric women than other women. Figure 8.1 also graphs the mean scores, according to age, of the entire adult female sample for stress arising from Exits and stress arising from other sources. From hereon, for reasons that will be explained later, the latter will be referred to as Miscellaneous Stress. As can be seen the occurrence of Miscellaneous Stress remains fairly constant over the entire female age range, whereas Exit Stress rises dramatically in the early climacteric, thereafter declining. Thus, the increase in Total Life Stress at the climacteric appears to be almost entirely accounted for by an increase in the number of persons leaving the woman's social field. This was thought to be an important finding, supporting the idea that certain life events occurring specifically at the time of the climacteric may have some special significance for certain women.

Specific Life Events

This hypothesis was further investigated by examining these two categories of life events to see whether or not any particular events were more frequent within each category, and to determine what precisely was accounting for the marked increase in Exits during the climacteric (Greene, 1982). It was first found that events contributing to Miscellaneous Stress were of a heterogeneous nature. Hence the use of the label Miscellaneous Stress to refer to this mixed group of events. Furthermore, there was, by and large, little variation between climacteric women and pre and postclimacteric women in regard to any particular event. The one exception to this was the occurrence of physical or emotional illness of a close family member *not* leading to death. This was almost twice as common among climacteric than preclimacteric women, accounting for about one-fifth of the life events in the miscellaneous category for the former. On the whole, however, recently occurring events making up the miscellaneous group were fairly commonplace ones, consisting of minor problems within the family, changes in work conditions, financial difficulties, housing inadequacies, minor illnesses and so on.

With regard to Exits, departures of others from the women's social field fell into three main categories — those due to children leaving home, those due to separation from another person and those due to deaths of a close friend, significant relative or family member (for clarification Figure 8.2 illustrates the categories into which all life events have been subdivided). Of the three categories of Exits, those due to *deaths* formed by far the *largest single group* among climacteric women, and accounted for some 60 per cent of all Exits among those women, as opposed to only 10 per cent in preclimacteric women.

This effect is illustrated in Figure 8.3, which shows that stress arising from deaths increases and peaks dramatically in the early part of the climacteric, and although declining in the latter part still remains substantially high. Deaths therefore, account almost entirely for the increase in Exit Stress during the entire climacteric, shown in Figure 8.1. Non-deaths Exits, that is separation from another person or the departure

```
                    ┌── Miscellaneous stress  (mainly minor and
                    │                          commonplace problems)
                    │
Total life stress ──┤                         ┌── Children leaving home
                    │                         │
                    │                         │
                    └── Exit stress ──────────┼── Separation from
                                              │   significant person
                                              │
                                              └── Deaths
```

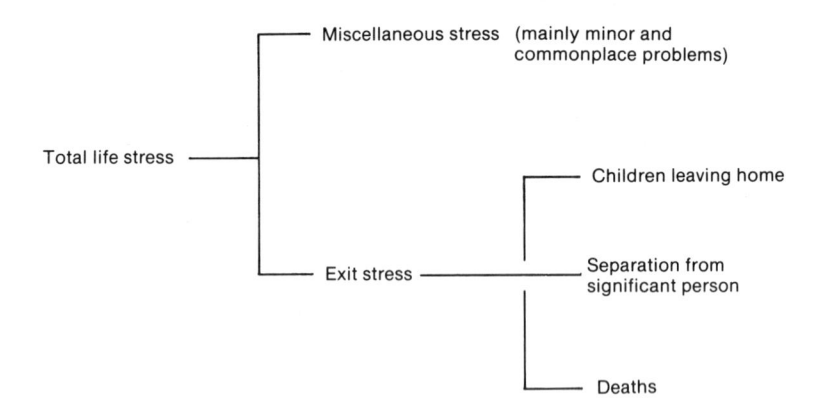

Figure 8.2 Schematic diagram of the main categories of life stress during the climacteric.

of a child, make up the rest of this total, and as can be seen this declines gradually over this age range. The increase in children leaving home during the climacteric was more than compensated for by a decline in the departure of other significant persons. Only one of the latter was the result of a marital break-up, the rest being mainly due to friends and family members moving to other areas.

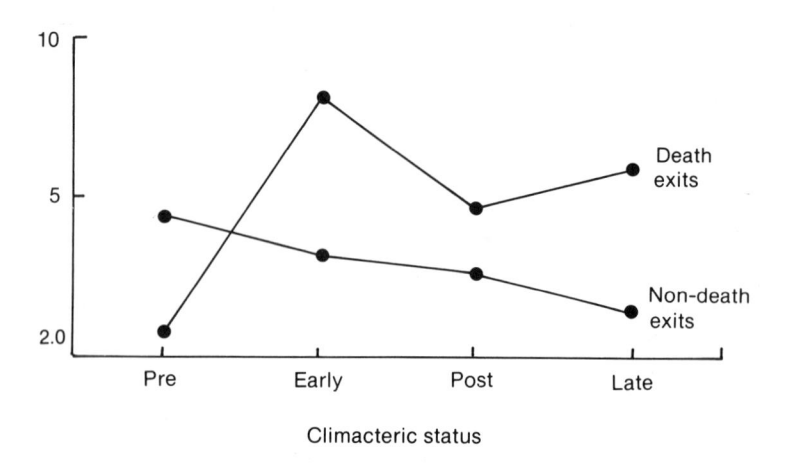

Figure 8.3 Mean stress scores for two subcategories of exits in relation to climacteric status.
(from Greene, 1982)

Types of Life Events and Symptoms

The relationships between symptoms and the three major categories into which Total Life Stress can be subdivided, namely, Miscellaneous Stress, Exits due to deaths and non-death Exits (separation and children leaving home) were then examined within the group of climacteric women (Greene, 1983). Considering non-death Exits first, these, as can be seen from Figure 8.3, were relatively low during the climacteric and were not found to be associated in any way with symptoms. This applied equally well to the subgroup of Exits involving children leaving home. These for the most part were for reasons of marriage, the great majority of which had parental approval. In the West of Scotland there is still a strong tendency for children to remain at home with their parents until the time of marriage. In the very few cases in which a child had left home without parental approval, among such women symptoms tended to be more frequent and severe. Clearly, what is important is the circumstances surrounding the departure of the child from home. A similar effect was noted by Lowenthal and Chiriboga (1972) in their longitudinal study of the effects of the 'empty nest' process on both men and women in the United States (see section 5.2).

Miscellaneous Stress, which included stress arising from commonplace problems, and which it will be recalled remained fairly constant over the entire female age range (see Figure 8.1), and stress arising from deaths were, however, associated with symptoms in a complex and interactive way, in which the effect of deaths on women depended on the level of Miscellaneous Stress they were experiencing. This effect can be best demonstrated by categorising women as to whether they were experiencing high or low levels of Miscellaneous Stress (this was done by dividing them at the median score) and as to whether they had experienced a death or not. Average total symptom scores for each of the four groups of women generated in this way are shown in Table 8.2. As can be seen, women experiencing a high level of Miscellaneous Stress show a high degree of symptomatology, an effect which is *heightened* in those women who have experienced a recent bereavement. In contrast, bereavement had no additional effect on symptoms in women reporting low levels of Miscellaneous Stress. Hence the interactive effect just referred to. Thus, symptoms were more severe among women experiencing many commonplace events and even moreso if, in addition, they had experienced a recent bereavement.

These results refer to total symptom scores. However, when somatic and psychological symptoms were examined separately, an interesting differential effect emerged. Corresponding results for somatic and

Table 8.2

Mean Total Symptoms Scores in
Relation to Miscellaneous Stress and Deaths

Death	Miscellaneous Stress	
	High	Low
Yes	22.48	11.33
No	15.25	11.75

From Greene (1983)

psychological symptoms are shown in Table 8.3. These reveal that the above interactive effect is much greater for somatic than psychological symptoms. That is, the increase in total symptom scores (Table 8.2) among those women experiencing both high levels of Miscellaneous

Table 8.3

Mean Scores on the Psychological and Somatic Symptom
Scales in Relation to Miscellaneous Stress and Deaths

Death	Miscellaneous Stress			
	High	Low	High	Low
Yes	14.45	7.5	8.03	3.83
No	11.67	8.5	3.58	3.25
	(Psychological)		(Somatic)	

Main effect of miscellaneous
stress on psychological symptoms, $P < 0.025$.
Interaction effect on somatic symptoms, $P < 0.05$.

From Greene (1983)

Stress and a recent bereavement, is due mostly, though not entirely, to an increase in physical complaints. Indeed, a stepwise multiple regression revealed that a significant interactive effect existed only in the case of somatic symptoms, there being a main effect only for Miscellaneous Stress on psychological symptoms. Thus, a high level of Miscellaneous

Stress alone is sufficient to produce an increase in psychological symptoms irrespective of the occurrence of a death. In the case of somatic symptoms neither a high degree of Miscellaneous Stress nor the occurrence of a death are in themselves sufficient. Both must be concomitantly high to produce an effect.

Bereavement During the Climacteric

Almost 40 per cent of this sample of Scottish climacteric women had reported experiencing in the year preceding the survey, the loss, through death, of a close friend, a significant relative or an immediate family member. The equivalent figure for preclimacteric women was 5 per cent. Bereavement was also fairly common among postclimacteric women in the age range 55 to 64 years, approximately one-third of whom had experienced such an event in the preceding year. These deaths were mostly of their own generation — husbands, siblings and contemporaries.

Deaths experienced by climacteric women, however, were mostly those of the older generation, being those of grandparents, parents, aunts and uncles, many of whom were reaching an age when the likelihood of illness and death increases. There was only one death of a spouse and none of children in the climacteric group. Furthermore, of those dying at least 70 per cent were described as having been a close friend, or of having played an important role in the life of the person. These details had been obtained at the time of interview, by means of a number of probe questions designed to assess the closeness of the woman's relationship with the deceased person. The significance of this additional finding will be outlined more fully in the next section.

8.3. DISCUSSION

The results of this study indicate that some of the increase in symptoms among this Scottish population of women at the climacteric, is associated with the degree of current life stress to which they become exposed at that time. The results also indicate that the relationship between symptoms and life events is not a simple one and that different types of symptoms are influenced by different types of life events in a complex and interactive way.

Psychological Symptoms

Consider first symptoms of a psychological nature. Among climacteric women, the increase in these symptoms at that time is directly related to the severity of Miscellaneous Life Stress. That is, the greater the total amount of stress arising from a variety of different sources — financial, legal, work, housing conditions, illness in the family, etc. — the greater are complaints of psychological symptoms. Yet this sort of life stress is not greater during the climacteric than at other times, nor are there any marked differences between preclimacteric and climacteric women in the sort of events giving rise to Miscellaneous Stress. These problems are very similar both in quality and quantity at both times of life and are of a fairly commonplace nature. The fact, therefore, that the increase in symptoms at the climacteric occurs mainly in women experiencing high levels of this Miscellaneous Stress, suggests that at that time women become less able to cope with problems with which at an earlier age they seem able to cope. Putting this another way, it suggests that during the climacteric some women become vulnerable to these sort of commonplace difficulties, and this vulnerability manifests itself mainly in the form of psychological complaints.

Somatic Symptoms

Somatic symptoms on the other hand, are also reported moreso by climacteric women who are experiencing high levels of Miscellaneous Stress, but *only* if they have also experienced a recent bereavement. These bereavements in themselves do not appear to have an effect on somatic symptoms, but do so only if women are currently experiencing stress from other sources. What seems to be happening is that the additional stress of bereavement 'adds on' mainly somatic symptoms to the existing psychological ones, among women already experiencing a high level of other types of stress. This can be seen by comparing Table 8.2 with Table 8.3.

There are two possible explanations for this effect. Firstly, it seems reasonable to suppose that this specific effect on somatic symptoms is in some way linked to the symptoms and illness of the deceased person. The effect may be further enhanced by the fact that women at this age may be experiencing age or hormone related physical changes, in which case illness and death of others may serve to exacerbate already existing somatic discomfort. Secondly, most of these deaths were described as being that of a person from the older generation with whom the women had a *close* supportive relationship. This suggests a possible reason as to why the effect on somatic symptoms occurs *only* in the presence of a high degree of Miscellaneous Stress. It suggests that this may not be a bereavement response per se, but rather that it is the consequences of the death that is critical. One of these consequences may be that these deaths deprive some of these women of the social and family support necessary for them to cope with their current difficulties.

Brown's Aetiological Model

How do these results and these putative explanations (vulnerability in climacteric women, somatisation of stress and loss of social support) relate to the findings and theories of other researchers in the field of life events? Probably the most comprehensive aetiological model of the relationship between life events and psychological disorder is that developed by the sociologist George Brown and his colleagues of Bedford College, London. This aetiological model was developed on the basis of community studies of the social origins of depression among women living in the London borough of Camberwell, a full description of which can be found in Brown and Harris (1978). This work however is not without its critics, notably Tennant and Bebbington (1978) who have criticised the methodology, conceptualisation of variables, mode of argument and statistical techniques employed in the analysis. This theoretical model is nevertheless relevant to the present author's findings in a number of ways and its key features will now be summarised.

Brown's method of eliciting and measuring life events has previously been described in section 8.1. In his theoretical model, life events, which are defined as discrete traumatic happenings occurring at a particular point in time (e.g. losing a job) are distinguished from ongoing difficulties, that may or may not have begun with a discrete incident (e.g. husband's unemployment or a son's alcoholism). Both are subsumed under the general heading of *provoking agents*, as factors capable of producing psychiatric illness. However, even if it was established that provoking agents and psychiatric illness were causally related, the question would arise as to why only some persons experiencing an event develop such an illness. This required the introduction of the notion of *vulnerability*. By definition, such factors are capable of increasing the risk of psychiatric illness only in the presence of a provoking agent. Alone, they have no effect at all. There is yet another set of factors in the model which influence illness, but unlike provoking agents and vulnerability factors, do not increase the risk of developing it. These are called *symptom formation* factors as they influence only the form and severity of the illness. These then are the three concepts central to Brown's aetiological model. For the remainder of this section we shall see how these can be used to interpret the present writer's findings.

Vulnerability at the Climacteric

In their study of the social origins of depression in Camberwell, Brown and his colleagues found that certain provoking agents, in this case severe events and major long term difficulties, were indeed capable of bringing about depression in women. Furthermore, the risk of depression in response to a provoking agent increased if, in addition, a woman had experienced certain background social factors. These vulnerability factors were, in the case of the Camberwell women, the presence of more than three children under 14 years in the household, the loss of a mother in childhood, the absence of a confiding relationship with her spouse and the lack of a job. The last two are of particular interest in view of the demonstrable effect poor marital relations and absence of employment outwith the home had on climacteric symptoms. These particular factors act only in the presence of a serious threat, that is a major provoking agent. However, in a later account, Brown et al. (1979) go onto consider 'further susceptibility factors that may increase the chance of depression irrespective of provoking agents as we define them' (p.210). Interestingly, in this context, they specifically refer to the role of ageing which they consider 'involves physiological changes but may also have psychosocial consequences which increase susceptibility such as, for example the mid-life crisis where depression may develop in response to *quite minor events*' (p.210, present author's italics).

It is not difficult to see the relevance of this quotation to the present author's results, where non-specific symptoms (which included some depressive ones) developed in climacteric women experiencing fairly commonplace life events arising from a number of sources — what has been called Miscellaneous Stress. Yet preclimacteric women do not develop such symptoms when exposed to similar amounts of this type of 'minor' stress. Unlike the work of Brown and his colleagues, the outcome measure was not serious psychiatric depression but a symptom scale containing common 'climacteric symptoms'. This difference in the outcome measure will be discussed later. At this point, however, there does seem to be some evidence from the present author's study in support of the conjecture of Brown et al. regarding climacteric women's greater vulnerability to life events.

Death as a Provoking Agent

Turning now from vulnerability to the nature of provoking agents, the study of the Bedford College group that is relevant here is not the Camberwell survey, but a more recent one carried out by this group in Scotland, this time in the Western Isles of Lewis and North Uist. This study was carried out, not only to test some of the hypotheses arising from the earlier research in Camberwell, but also, to extend ideas about the aetiology of affective disorders. A full account of this study is given in Brown and Prudo (1981) and Prudo et al. (1981).

The most striking difference between the London and Western Isles studies was the prominent role played by bereavement as a provoking agent of psychiatric disorders among the Scottish women. In all, 48 per cent of onset depressive cases in the Hebrides were preceded by a severe event, involving death or clear intimation of a death of a close relative, compared with only 16 per cent of London women. The fact that such events were not more common in the Hebrides than London, led the authors to conclude that Hebridean women are particularly sensitive to death or imminent death of a close relative. Not only did a greater proportion of Hebridean than London women develop depression following events involving death in the year of the study, but these events played a major role in bringing abut the *chronicity* of different types of psychiatric conditions at the case and borderline case levels of severity in the Hebrides. Indeed, 77 per cent of all chronic psychiatric disorders in the Hebrides had been provoked by the death of a close relative compared with only 16 per cent in Camberwell. Although events involving death clearly constitute provoking agents in the Brown aetiological model, these authors consider that the greater sensitivity of Hebridean women to death might be more parsimoniously incorporated into their concept of vulnerability.

Cultural Sensitivity to Death

Brown and his colleagues attribute this heightened sensitivity to family deaths to the type and degree of attachments Hebridean women have to relatives, especially to members of their 'natal' family, i.e. their family of origin. This they in turn attribute to certain traditional sociocultural aspects of Hebridean society, which may operate on women at different levels, both sociological and psychological. A full account of this is provided in the discussion section of Prudo et al. (1981). Suffice it here however, to emphasise that the critical losses are those of members of the women's *natal* family, that is parents, aunts, uncles and siblings. These are thought to be critical because of the extraordinary strong kinship bonds and the wide prevalence of the extended family household in the Hebrides. This is a consequence of a system of agriculture and croft ownership, in which kin are still paramount.

Again it is not difficult to see parallels between Brown's findings in the Hebrides and the present author's findings in the sample of urban climacteric Scottish women. The common element, of course, is the degree of these Scottish women's sensitivity to the death of friends and members of their natal family. It will be recalled that the majority of deaths experienced by Glasgow women at the climacteric were exactly those of such persons. But here the parallels seem to end, as such deaths elicit psychiatric depression in Hebridean women, and merely common climacteric symptoms, with a strong somatic component, in urban climacteric women.

Deaths and Climacteric Symptoms

A relevant finding in the Hebridean study was the high degree of occurrence of anxiety and phobic disorders among women following the loss of someone close. This led the authors to conclude that events involving death played 'a major role in bringing about the chronicity of depressive and *anxiety or phobic* disorders at the case and *borderline* case levels of severity' (p.610, present author's italics). Furthermore, the type of relative lost was related to the form of symptoms. Those losing a parent 'were most likely to have an anxiety or phobic disorder, and those losing other close relatives (husband or child) a depressive disorder' (p.610). This therefore, provides a further link between the two studies as it will be recalled that among climacteric women, of all deaths, only one was of a husband and none was of a child and the symptoms were of a psychosomatic/anxiety type (palpitations, dizzy spells, breathlessness etc.).

Why should deaths of natal family members (parents, aunts, uncles, siblings) provoke a specific phobic anxiety reaction in these women? Brown and his colleagues again account for this in terms of the well defined, but rigid, role women occupy in the tightly knit Hebridean social network. This role makes a woman strongly identify with and be dependent on her natal family. Because of the limited nature of this role, these deaths seriously undermine a woman's 'role identity', and for this reason they are perceived, in Brown's terminology, as a 'danger'. This 'danger' elicits a psychologically primitive emotional response such as those of anxiety and phobic symptoms. For a fuller account of this life event model of anxiety see Finlay-Jones and Brown (1981).

The response of most Glaswegian climacteric women to deaths of natal family members is nonetheless less severe than that of Hebridean women and is marked by a strong somatic component. The reasons for this less severe reaction may be that the sensitivity of Glasgow women to these deaths of close relatives is somewhat less than that of Hebridean women, although the reasons for their sensitivity may be similar. The part of the city from which these women come, contains large pockets of working class populations. In these areas traditional Scottish working class attitudes and values still prevail. These populations are essentially immobile, and within them remnants of the extended family and strong familial bonds still exist. The role of women in the system also still has strong traditional aspects. This type of culture could be regarded as not dissimilar in many ways to that existing in the Hebrides, although being in an urban region it is clearly much less traditional and closed. The predominance of somatic symptoms in their reaction is presumably linked to the death of their relative, either in the form of an 'incorporation' of the deceased's symptoms and illness, or else in the form of an exacerbation of concomitant physical climacteric and age related symptoms.

Loss of Social Support

The foregoing provides a possible explanation for the relatively high degree of sensitivity of this sample of Glaswegian women to death. But why does this sensitivity manifest itself among climacteric women *only* in the presence of other stress? (see Table 8.3). One of the consequences of the death of a relative or friend with whom one has had a close relationship is the loss of that person's help and support at times of crisis. Indeed, one of the major vulnerability factors predisposing women to depression in the Camberwell study was the lack of a close intimate relationship with their spouse (Brown and Harris, 1978). There is also evidence from other life event research work as to the importance of supportive relationships of this type in protecting individuals from stress (Cobb, 1976; Paykel et al., 1980; Henderson, 1981).

The work which provides strongest support for this explanation, however, is that of the Medical Research Council Epidemiology Unit at the Royal Edinburgh Hospital in Scotland. Miller and Ingham (1976) and Miller et al. (1976) found that among a group of patients consulting a general practice with minor psychological and physical symptoms, both having few acquaintances and not having a confidant, were related to high symptom levels, particularly psychological symptoms, and *particularly in women*. Another link between that study and the present one is these authors' conclusion regarding the relationship between life events and different types of symptoms. On the basis of their results Miller et al. (1976) postulate that 'people's first reaction to stressful life events is psychological; and that if life events are *linked to physical ailments* these latter are the result of, or are exacerbated by, the initial anxiety, depression etc., if it lasts long enough' (p.521, present author's italics).

This concurs with the present author's suggestion regarding the somatisation of complaints among climacteric women in response to deaths. Among climacteric women experiencing natal family deaths, these events are not only linked to the woman's own physical complaints at that time, but they are also linked to the illness and symptoms of the deceased person. It should also be noted that the physical symptoms referred to by Miller et al. (1976) are identical to those included in the Climacteric Symptom Rating scale constructed by the present author — backache, headaches, palpitations, dizziness, breathlessness — all of which could be considered to be of a psychogenic nature. It also follows that the loss of such support in adversity would, a priori, be even greater among Scottish climacteric women, in view of the close nature of their family ties, as sensitivity to natal family deaths and loss of social support must be intimately related.

Conclusion

The aetiological model proposed here, linking life events of recent onset to symptoms among Scottish climacteric women, has close parallels to that of Brown and his colleagues regarding psychiatric disorders in Hebridean women. To begin with, the climacteric period per se may act as a vulnerability factor, in that 'quite minor events' (Brown's words) in the form of Miscellaneous Stress, may provoke symptoms to a greater degree at that time of life than at other times. Moreover, for this particular group of climacteric women, if the death of a natal family member occurs at the same time, this acts as an additional provoking agent. The potency of this provoking agent for these particular women is explained in terms of cultural sensitivity to such deaths, which serves as a vulnerability factor. Deaths, or more precisely the illness and symptoms of the now deceased person, also act as symptom formation factors by exacerbating somatic symptoms among women already experiencing somatic discomfort for hormonal and other reasons. However, as somatic symptoms are

Provoking Agent
(miscellaneous or
minor stress;
deaths)

Vulnerability Factors
(being climacteric;
sensitivity to natal
deaths; loss of social
support)

Symptom Formation Factors
(illness, symptoms of deceased)

The Climacteric Syndrome
— Psychological symptoms
— Somatic symptoms

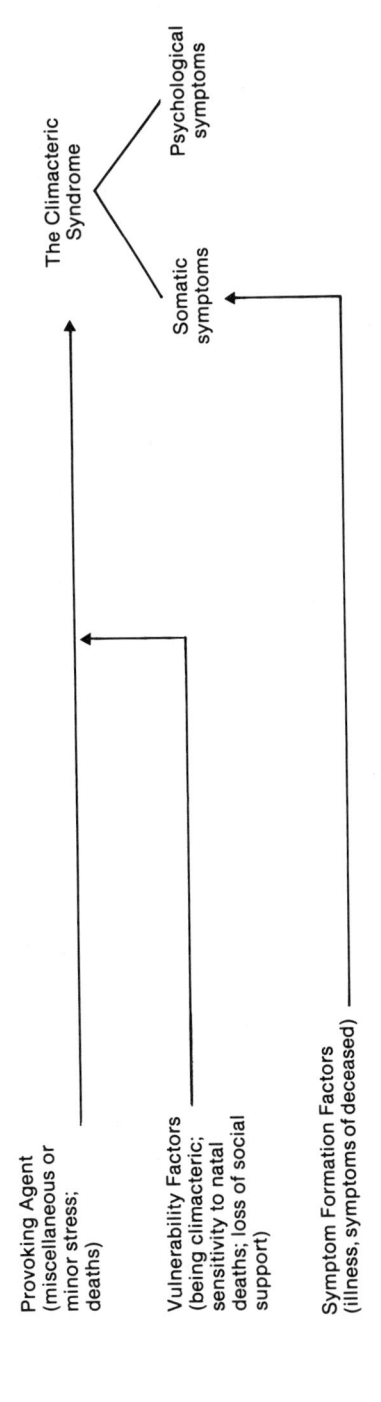

Figure 8.4 Schematic diagram of relationship between life events and climacteric symptoms in a sample of urban Scottish women, using Brown's terminology.

exacerbated only in women experiencing high levels of Miscellaneous Stress, a fourth element is hypothesised by which deaths act to make climacteric women even more vulnerable. This is by depriving those climacteric women, currently experiencing minor stress, of a source of social support at a time when they particularly need such support.

This model, in which the element of specific cultural sensitivity is incorporated into the more general climacteric vulnerability to minor life events, is schematically represented in Figure 8.4, using Brown's terminology. There it can be seen that all recently occurring life events (Miscellaneous Stress and deaths) are depicted as provoking agents for symptoms among climacteric women. Being climacteric is grouped under vulnerability factors, as minor life events provoke symptoms to a greater extent at that time of life. Sensitivity to natal family deaths is similarly classified, since somatic symptoms are produced in response to deaths to a greater degree, if such sensitivity exists either within a culture or an individual. Loss of social support is also classified as a vulnerability factor as deaths have a greater effect in the presence of a high level of Miscellaneous Stress. In any case loss of social support and sensitivity to natal family deaths are obviously intimately related. Finally, the illness and symptoms of the deceased person are classified as symptom formation factors because of their specific role in provoking additional somatic symptoms.

The causal model outlined in Figure 8.4 is not intended to be a fully comprehensive or definitive one of the link between life events and climacteric symptoms. Its object is merely to account for the empirical relationships found in this particular sample of Scottish climacteric women using Brown's terminology. There may in fact be other types of life event relationships which have not emerged in this study. Nor is it in any way intended to explain *all* symptoms among *all* climacteric women.

9

A Vulnerability Model of the Climacteric

In this monograph I have been primarily concerned with examining the relevant research literature for evidence as to how, and to what extent, sociocultural and psychological factors influence the responses and experiences of women during the climacteric phase of their lives. In doing this, a fairly wide concept of the climacteric and what constitutes the climacteric syndrome has been adopted. This has been based on the set of definitions drawn up by Utian and Serr (1976), a set of definitions which have become generally accepted by most researchers in this field. In this system, climacteric symptoms are considered to arise from three main sources — decreased ovarian activity, sociocultural and psychological factors. In this final chapter, I shall draw together the diverse material which has emerged in the preceding chapers, and in doing so, attempt to arrive at a comprehensive but cohesive sociopsychological model of the climacteric syndrome based on the available research. Before doing this I shall briefly summarise the contribution the first of these sources makes to the climacteric syndrome. Throughout this chapter, figures in parentheses refer to the relevant sections of this volume.

The Contribution of Oestrogen Deficiency

At the outset, it was seen how diverse clinical opinion was regarding which of the many symptoms occurring during the climacteric period, could be attributed to the effects of oestrogen deficiency (2.1), despite the fact that the only symptoms, which there were sound reasons for believing could be so explained, were those of vasomotor instability and atrophic vaginitis (1.2). Furthermore, a close examination of the outcome of clinical trials of oestrogen therapy convincingly demonstrated that there was very little reason for supposing that symptoms, other than the latter, can be alleviated by oestrogen replacement, over and above a placebo or a domino effect, arising from the relief of vasomotor symptoms and those of atrophic vaginitis (2.3). In particular the notion that oestrogen has a specific psychotropic effect was discounted in the light of the evidence (2.4).

In later chapters vasomotor symptoms also stood out as being quite different from others in their close temporal association with the menopause (3.2), in being essentially unrelated to sociodemographic factors (5.3), in their stability across cultures (3.2 and 6.2), in their lack of association with other symptoms in both cluster and factor analytic studies (3.2 and 7.4) and in their immunity from the effects of stressful life events (8.2). However, in those chapters, many of the variables found to be unassociated with vasomotor symptoms did exercise an effect on the other symptoms, especially the psychological ones, which make up the climacteric syndrome. This has given rise to a wealth of both positive and negative findings. The problem now is one of subsuming this variety of psychological, sociological and anthropological findings within a comprehensive, but parsimonious, explanatory framework.

Climacteric Vulnerability

One way of starting this exercise is to begin with the notion of vulnerability. That is, to see the climacteric as a time of life when women may become more likely to display signs of physical, psychological and social distress. As we have seen, there is good evidence that as well as there being an increase in what we have chosen to call non-specific symptomatology during the climacteric (3.2), there is also a decline in certain other aspects of psychological and social functioning (4.1 and 4.2). These effects could, ipso facto, be taken as reflecting the general vulnerability of women at the time, presumably because they are passing through a critical transitional phase of their lives (1.3).

However, to begin with, climacteric vulnerability does not seem to operate in a simple direct causal manner. Many of the characteristics and functions adversely affected during the climacteric are also at the same time declining with age, or may represent the accentuation of an existing problem or the recurrence of an earlier one. All three of these effects apply to sexual difficulties (4.2), the first to the IHF measure, of Subjective Adaptation (4.1) and the third to formal psychiatric disorders (4.3), should they occur during the climacteric. All three may also apply, in varying degrees, to symptoms (3.2). Thus, the climacteric does not seem to act as a primary vulnerability factor per se, but acts to *accentuate* an already existing problem, *accelerate* the effects of ageing or cause previous problems to *recur*. Nor, given the modest magnitude of the increase in, for example, non-specific, in contrast to the large increase in vasomotor symptoms, can these effects act equally on all women to the same extent. This raises the question of whether we can identify those women, or those groups of women, who, during the climacteric are more vulnerable than others. The answer to this question seems to be very definite 'yes'.

Factors Determining Vulnerability

Throughout Chapters 5 and 6 it was clearly and consistently demonstrated that it was, what one might call, *underprivileged* women who suffered most during the climacteric. By this is meant, those of low social class, of low family income, of low educational level (5.3), as well as those living in arduous and culturally deprived environments (6.2). Women who had no occupation outwith the home were also more vulnerable, but this too was associated with being underprivileged, since being employed had a protective effect only if the woman was of higher social class or pursuing a professional career, and had a detrimental effect if otherwise (5.3). Furthermore, there was some evidence that the above mentioned accentuation, acceleration and recurrence effects on symptoms and other functions, tended to occur predominately among women of low socioeconomic class (5.3). The responses of these less privileged women seem to be mediated, in part at least, by socially determined attitudes to the menopause, since women of lower social class have a consistently negative stereotype of that event and its consequences (6.1). In short, the effect at the climacteric of being socially disadvantaged is a profound and widespread one.

Moreover, when more personal and individual circumstances were examined, it was found that it was women with pre-existing problems or long standing difficulties, such as marital dissatisfaction, problems in early development, financial and economic difficulties, who reacted most adversely during the climacteric (5.2). Strangely, there was little evidence to support the hypothesis that those changes thought to be peculiar to the mid-life period contributed much to distress during the climacteric. Most notable of these was the failure to find any adverse effects arising from the departure of children from home (5.2).

This was also apparent in the author's study of life events during the climacteric, in which it was found that most of the recent onset events provoking symptoms were of a minor and commonplace sort, and were found with equal frequency among younger women (8.2). In contrast, however, younger women experiencing these same events during the preclimacteric, showed no such excess of symptoms. This again underpoints the vulnerability of climacteric women. In that study, the events found to be especially critical during the climacteric were deaths of natal family members, but as reactions to these were thought to be culturally specific, these will be discussed more fully, later in this chapter.

The significance of the loss of reproductive function also features highly in the climacteric literature and there was some evidence that loss of the reproductive role may have an effect on women's attitudes to the menopause, if this role is a highly valued one (6.1). This must however be viewed in the context of the social structure of the particular society, thereby necessitating a consideration of comparative studies of cultural influences, as there are good reasons for believing that these influences are highly diverse (6.2). This raises the question of the mechanism whereby socioeconomic and cultural factors exercise their influence.

Alternative Social Roles

As a general rule, women's attitudes to the menopause in different cultures are based to a large extent on the perceived consequences it has for their social role and status. Whether this attitude will be a predominately negative one will depend on the extent to which that event is seen as adversely affecting their position in society. This effect, it would seem, is determined by three factors. These are, the social structure and cultural mores of the society, socioeconomic factors and at what stage the society is in the transition from being a traditional to a modern one (6.3). The common element linking these three factors may be whether or not there exists within a society recognised alternative roles for the postreproductive women. Considering the last factor first, we have seen how, as a society moves along this traditional modern continuum, women become more preoccupied with the psychological and social consequences of the menopause and less with the reproductive and physical ones (6.2). This clearly reflects the centrality of the child bearing and rearing roles in traditional societies and its decreasing importance as this continuum is traversed.

Furthermore, it would appear that women in societies which are in the middle of this transition suffer more during the climacteric than do those living in more modern or traditional cultures. It is hypothesised that this is because in those traditional societies which are passing through a transitional phase, women in general may not as yet have developed alternative and appropriate roles or outlets, once the reproductive phase of their lives had ceased. This is particularly so if the process of 'acculturation' has been a rapid one. In some stable traditional societies, the tight social networks, and in particular the family system, provide for a natural and gradual role transition at the climacteric. In others, it may be that the negative social consequences of the menopause are mitigated by the establishment of special compensatory roles or functions, such as occur in some North American Indian tribes, in which the postmenopausal women may aspire to the role of someone with supernatural powers (6.2). Such roles may have disappeared in cultures passing through the transitional phase. In this context, Griffen (1982) has suggested that where there is no cultural agreement on the role or status of the postmenopausal women, or even an agreement that her status is an anomalous one, tension develops around her role. Therefore, in those societies in which the stereotype of the menopause is a negative one, or in which its consequences are negatively evaluated and in which there exist no established postreproductive roles, the effect of the climacteric on women will be most adverse.

Alternative Roles and Socioeconomic Status

The availability of alternative social roles may apply equally well within modern pluralistic societies, as to more traditional ones, and may help explain some of the variation in response during the climacteric within modern societies in which responses have been shown to be less uniform (6.2). It may explain, for example, why women of low socioeconomic status in Western societies react so adversely during the climacteric (5.3). In these societies, although in some respects women of low socioeconomic status have adopted more contemporary attitudes, for example, with regard to their reproductive role, in other respects they still occupy a more traditional one. Certainly the negative stereotype of the menopause held by these women seems to be based on a more traditional conception of the female role in society (6.1). They, like women in some traditional societies, could be seen as passing through a 'transitional phase' in which satisfactory alternative postreproductive social roles have not as yet been fully developed. Women of high socioeconomic status and educational level, on the other hand, have been able to develop such roles and therefore do not see the climacteric as heralding the cessation of their social usefulness and status.

This of course, could also account for the protective nature of employment outwith the home (5.3), as this clearly facilitates women to develop alternative roles. Moreover, merely being occupied outwith the home is not enough, since if the woman is of lower social class, employment has no protective effect and may indeed be detrimental. In this context Warr (1983), on the basis of extensive research into the psychology of employment, has distinguished between what he calls psychologically 'good' and psychologically 'bad' jobs. The features of the latter is that they contain less variety, less goals, less decision making latitude, less skill, less interpersonal contact and less valued social position than the former. Such jobs, according to Warr, impair psychological wellbeing. Clearly the sort of jobs available to middle aged women of low socioeconomic status and educational level would be of this kind. What seems to be required is that the work be of a nature which enables the postmenopausal women to make a personally gratifying and socially significant contribution. Thus the principle determining variation *between* societies, namely the existence of alternative social roles, may also help account for some of the variations *within* societies, in women's responses during the climacteric.

Specific Cultural Sensitivity

Deaths of members of the older generation, particularly parents, is another set of events often quoted as exercising an important influence on women during the climacteric period (5.1). As deaths of such persons at that time of life, are not generally premature, a severe bereavement reaction would be unlikely to be a common response. However, we saw in Chapter 8 an example of what could be interpreted as a case of cultural specificity in vulnerability to such deaths among women living in a modern pluralistic society, namely, the United Kingdom. Sensitivity to deaths of natal family (the family of one's origin) was found to be a factor in predisposing women living in an urban Scottish community to develop climacteric symptoms, should such deaths occur at that time (8.2.).

This degree of sensitivity to these deaths was thought to be a cultural phenomenon, an interpretation based on the work of the sociologist George Brown. Brown and his colleagues had found wide differences between Scottish Hebridean women, on the one hand, and women living in London on the other, in their reactions to deaths of natal family members. These authors attributed the greater sensitivity of Hebridean women to these deaths, to the close supportive kinship bonds existing in that rural island community (8.3).

A similar interpretation was placed by the present author on the responses of the group of Scottish climacteric women to such deaths, despite their living in an urban community. The reasons being that traditional attitudes, values and family structures are still to be found in many Scottish communities, whether they be rural or urban, especially among working class populations. This cultural sensitivity to deaths of natal family members led to an exacerbation of somatic climacteric symptoms, but only among women who were at the same time experiencing psychological stress arising from a number of other life problems. This specific cultural vulnerability had therefore, to be incorporated into the more general life event vulnerability model of the climacteric, the central feature of which is that quite minor events may provoke psychological, and to a lesser degree physical symptoms to a greater extent among climacteric women, than women of other ages. In incorporating sensitivity to deaths into this model, other life event research concepts were utilised. Thus such deaths were also seen, by provoking somatic symptoms, to act as symptom formation factors, and also served to deprive these women, because of the closeness of the kinship bonds, of the social support necessary to counter current adversity. This model is summarised in the conclusion of section 8.3 and schematically depicted in Figure 8.4.

It is not, of course, being suggested that sensitivity to natal family deaths is a universal phenomenon among climacteric women. Whether it occurs or not will depend on the familial and social structure of a particular society or, as we have seen in this intance, subculture of a society.

Self-Esteem

To explain how vulnerability factors operate at the level of the individual to render a woman more sensitive to provoking agents, Brown and Harris (1978) introduce the concept of self-esteem. This is defined as feelings of low self-worth and inability to control events, leading to a sense of helplessness in the face of adversity. The various pre-existing vulnerability factors act to induce this psychological state, thereby rendering a woman less able to cope with stressful life events and therefore more likely to develop symptoms and psychiatric illness in response to their occurrence.

It is not difficult to see how two of Brown's vulnerability factors, lack of a confiding relationship with spouse and lack of employment outwith the home, may induce such a psychological state of mind. Self-esteem, in the sense of self-worth, is invariably derived from gratifying relationships, which provide the individual with what is called role identity. Thus Brown and Harris (1978) write:

> In the case of employment, not only does the role identity of worker become available to a woman but her extra social contacts will often provide her with new interpersonal identities. The existence of an intimate relationship most probably acts by providing not only role identity but also one that is likely to be appraised as successful and thus a source of self-esteem (p.237).

One of these vulnerability factors, lack of intimacy, in the form of poor marital relations, has been shown to be implicated in negative reactions during the climacteric (5.2). The other, being employed, the absence of which has featured prominently as being associated with climacteric symptoms in this volume (5.3), has been identified by Ginsberg (1976) as a source of self-esteem for women in general, within any society where status accrues to economic gain, and by Kaufert (1982) as a possible source of self-esteem for climacteric women in particular. Another of Brown's vulnerability factors, specific cultural sensitivity to death, was also a feature of Scottish climacteric women (8.3). This vulnerability factor exercises its effect by disrupting the close kinship bonds and family ties from which these women derive much of their role identity and therefore self-esteem. Thus, self-esteem can be seen, at the level of the individual to be the mediator between, on the one hand, the subjective symptomatic and other responses women exhibit during the climacteric, and the various pre-existing vulnerability factors on the other. The concepts of vulnerability and reduced self-esteem carry with them the implication that such women may be at risk at other critical phases of the life cycle, such as adolescence and old age.

Conclusion

The concept of vulnerability would seem to be a useful and parsimonious one with which to account for the wide variability, both within and between societies in women's responses and experiences during the climacteric. It has been used in the foregoing discussion in many ways. To begin with, the climacteric period of life per se has been depicted as a vulnerable time of life, at least for some women, in that already existing problems may be accentuated, old ones made to recur and the psychological effects of ageing accelerated. In addition some women may find it increasingly difficult to cope with minor commonplace stress occurring at that time. However, we have also seen how the effects of climacteric vulnerability can be further exacerbated (or modified) by broadly based sociodemographic and sociocultural factors. It is hypothesised that these exercise their effect mainly by the extent to which they either promote or prevent postmenopausal women from developing personally satisfying and socially significant roles. This vulnerability may be further contributed to by the adverse effects of personal and social difficulties, predating the climacteric. Finally, the influences of life events and coincidental stresses which have their onset at some time during the climacteric, and whose effects are also mediated by vulnerability factors (see Figure 8.4) must be incorporated into this overall vulnerability model. Thus, in this model the concept of vulnerability acts throughout as a major cohesive factor.

This general vulnerability model is set out schematically in Figure 9. There, under 'mechanism of effect', the ways in which symptoms and other social and psychological functions (the dependent variables), are affected during the climacteric by the independent or aetiological variables, are depicted. These effects are exacerbated by the various predisposing factors, mediated by self-esteem. Decreased ovarian activity, although having its primary effect on vasomotor symptoms, has also been depicted as having an indirect influence on the dependent variables, mediated in this case by 'physiological instability'.

We conclude on two important points. The first is that the above vulnerability model leans heavily on concepts derived from life event research. It is not however, being suggested that this in any way represents a definitive nor universal model of the social and psychological origins of the climacteric experience. These concepts have been used merely as a convenient way of structuring the currently available empirical evidence. The content (that is, the variables shown in brackets in Figure 9), as opposed to the structure of this model will clearly depend on the nature of the sociocultural and socioeconomic milieu of a particular society.

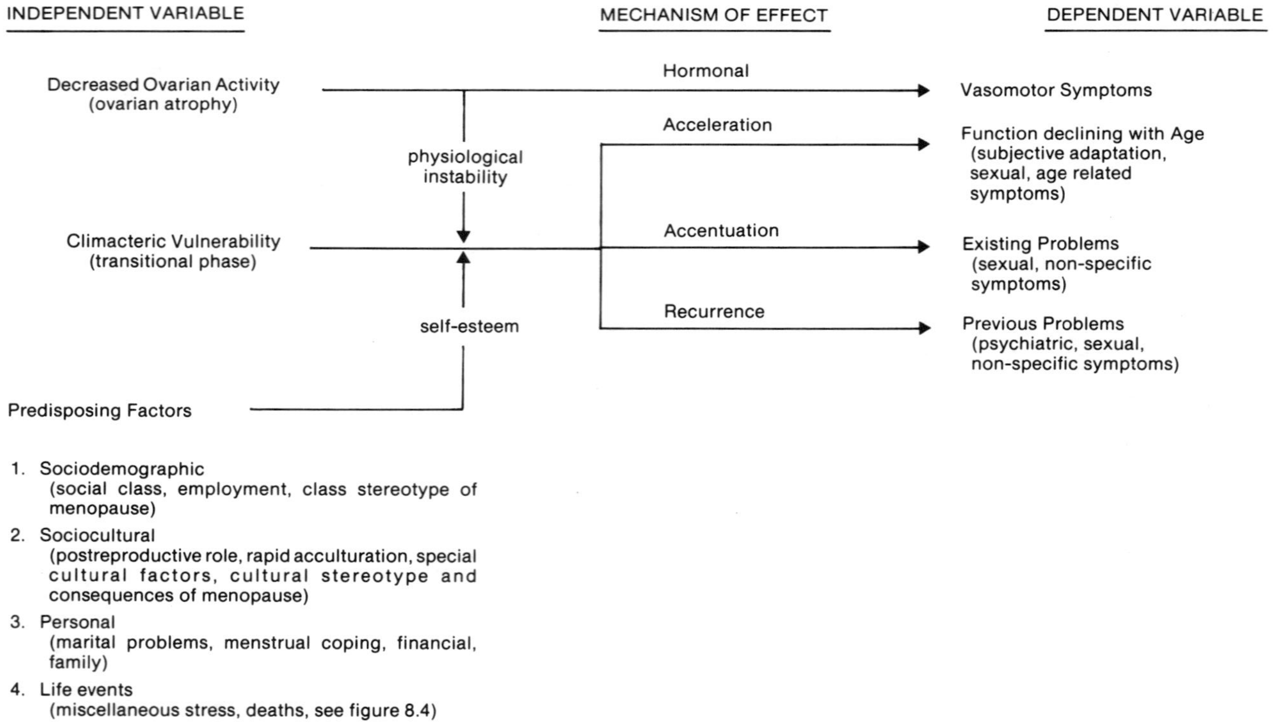

INDEPENDENT VARIABLE	MECHANISM OF EFFECT	DEPENDENT VARIABLE
Decreased Ovarian Activity (ovarian atrophy)	Hormonal → Acceleration	Vasomotor Symptoms
	Accentuation	Function declining with Age (subjective adaptation, sexual, age related symptoms)
Climacteric Vulnerability (transitional phase)	Recurrence	Existing Problems (sexual, non-specific symptoms)
		Previous Problems (psychiatric, sexual, non-specific symptoms)

physiological instability → ← self-esteem

Predisposing Factors

1. Sociodemographic (social class, employment, class stereotype of menopause)
2. Sociocultural (postreproductive role, rapid acculturation, special cultural factors, cultural stereotype and consequences of menopause)
3. Personal (marital problems, menstrual coping, financial, family)
4. Life events (miscellaneous stress, deaths, see figure 8.4)

Figure 9 A vulnerability model of the climacteric

Indeed, in other cultures and social subgroups other vulnerability factors, life events and personal circumstances may prove to be of relatively greater significance. We have seen, for example, in the study by Holte and Mikkelsen (1982) how socioeconomic factors, which in most studies have been found to exercise a profound effect on psychological symptom, had little such effect on Norwegian women, whereas more personal factors had a greater influence. This lack of effect was thought to be due to the socioeconomic homogeneity of Scandinavian society.

What is being argued is that the process or mechanics may be universal and that the theoretical concepts and methods of life event research provide a fruitful framework within which to investigate and conceptualise these causal relationships. As was stated in the introduction to Chapter 8, it is only by employing established conceptual and methodological frameworks of this type, that climacteric research can be brought into the mainstream of contemporary social science research and thinking.

The second point on which we conclude is that this vulnerability model appears to emphasise the negative side of the climacteric. This is not necessarily the case. The opposite of vulnerability factors is not merely their absence. Their opposite is the presence of positive factors, such as satisfactory employment opportunities, high status postreproductive roles, positive attitudes to the menopause, confiding and supportive relationships, positive life events, and so on; all of which lead to *high* self-esteem. It is perhaps this side of the coin that should be emphasised more, because it is by ensuring these, that the style and quality of life of the postreproductive woman will in the future be as it ought.

Bibliography

Adelstein, A., Downham, D. and Stein, Z. (1968) The epidemiology of mental illness in an English city. *Social Psychiatry*, vol. 3, pp. 47-59.
Aksel, S., Schomberg, D., Tyrey, L. and Hammond, C. (1976) Vasomotor symptoms, serum estrogens and gonadotrophin levels in surgical menopause. *American Journal of Obstetrics and Gynecology*, vol. 126, pp. 165-9.
American Psychiatric Association (1968) *Diagnostic and Statistical Manual of Mental Disorders*. Second Edition. APA, Washington.
Amundsen, D. and Diers, C. (1973) The age of menopause in mediaeval Europe. *Human Biology*, vol. 45, pp. 605-12.
Anastasi, A. (1976) *Psychological Testing*. Macmillan, New York.
Andrews, G. and Tennant, C. (1978) Editorial: Life event stress and psychiatric illness. *Psychological Medicine*, vol. 8, pp. 545-9.
Aylward, M. (1973) Plasma tryptophan levels and mental depression in postmenopausal subjects: Effects of oral piperazine — oestrone sulphate. *International Research Communications System*, vol. 1, p. 30.

Aylward, M., Holly, F. and Parker, R.J. (1974) An evaluation of clinical response to piperazine oestrone sulphate (Harmogen) in menopausal patients. *Current Medical Research and Opinion*, vol. 2, pp. 417-23.

Ballinger, C.B. (1975) Psychiatric morbidity and the menopause: Screening of general population sample. *British Medical Journal*, vol. 3, pp. 344-6.

Ballinger, C.B. (1976) Psychiatric morbidity and the menopause: Clinical features. *British Medical Journal*, vol. 1, pp. 1183-5.

Ballinger, C.B. (1977) Psychiatric moribidity and the menopause: Survey of a gynaecological out-patient clinic. *British Journal of Psychiatry*, vol. 131, pp. 83-9.

Bancroft, J. (1978) The relationship between hormones and sexual behaviour, in J.B. Hutchinson (ed.), *Biological Determinants of Behaviour*. Wiley, New York.

Bancroft, J. (1980) The endocrinology of sexual function. *Clinics in Obstetrics and Gynaecology*, vol. 7, pp. 253-81.

Bart, P. (1969) Why women's status changes in middle age. *Sociological Symposium*, vol. 3, pp. 1-18.

Bart, P. (1971) Depression in middle-aged women, in V. Gornick and B. Moran (eds.), *Woman in Sexist Society*. Basic Books, New York.

Bart, P. and Grossman, M. (1978) Menopause, in M. Notman and C. Nadelson (eds.), *The Woman Patient: Medical and Psychological Interfaces*. Plenum Press, New York.

Beard, R.J. (1976) *Menopause - Guide to Current Research and Practice*. MTP Press, Lancaster.

Beck, A., Ward, C., Mendelson, M., Mock, J. and Erbaugh, J. (1961) An inventory for measuring depression. *Archives of General Psychiatry*, vol. 4, pp. 561-71.

Blatt, M.H., Wiesbader, H. and Kupperman, H.S. (1953) Vitamin E and climacteric symptoms. *Archives of Internal Medicine*, vol. 91, pp. 792-9.

Block, E. (1952) Quantitative morphological investigations of the follicular system in women: Variations at different ages. *Acta Anatomica*, vol. 14, pp. 108-23.

Bodnar, S. and Catterill, T.B. (1972) Amitriptyline in emotional states associated with the climacteric. *Psychosomatics*, vol. 13, pp. 117-9.

Bolding, O.T. and Willicut, H. (1969) Physiological and psychological evaluation of the estrogen deprived patient. *Journal of the Medicine Association of Alabama*, vol. 39, p. 459-63.

Bottiglioni, F. and De Aloysio, D. (1982) Female sexual activity as a function of climacteric conditions and age. *Maturitas*, vol. 4, pp. 27-32.

Brand, P. (1978) *Age at Menopause*. Elve Labor Vincit, Leiden.
Brooks-Gunn, J. (1982) A sociocultural approach, in A. Voda, M. Dinnerstein and S. O'Donnell (eds.), *Changing Perspectives on Menopause*. University of Texas Press, Austin.
Brown, G.W. (1972) Life events and psychiatric illness: Some thoughts on methodology and causality. *Journal of Psychosomatic Research*, vol. 16, pp. 311-20.
Brown, G.W. (1981) Life events, psychiatric disorder and physical illness. *Journal of Psychosomatic Research*, vol. 25, pp. 461-73.
Brown, G.W. and Harris, T. (1978) *The Social Origins of Depression: A Study of Psychiatric Disorder in Women*. Tavistock, London.
Brown, G.W., Ni Bhrolchain, M. and Harris, T.O. (1979) Psychotic and neurotic depression: Aetiological and background factors. *Journal of Affective Disorders*, vol. 1, pp. 195-211.
Brown, G.W. and Prudo, R. (1981) Psychiatric disorder in a rural and an urban population: 1. Aetiology of depression. *Psychological Medicine*, vol. 11, pp. 581-99.
Brown, G.W., Sklair, F., Harris, T. and Birley, J.L. (1973) Life events and psychiatric disorder: 2. Some methodological issues. *Psychological Medicine*, vol. 3, pp. 74-87.
Bungay, G., Vessay, M. and McPherson, C. (1980) Study of symptoms in middle life with special reference to the menopause. *British Medical Journal*, vol. 281, pp. 181-3.
Burch, P. and Gunz, F. (1967) The distribution of menopausal age in New Zealand. An exploratory study. *New Zealand Medical Journal*, vol. 66, pp. 6-10.
Campagnoli, C., Morra, G., Belforte, P., Belforte, L. and Tousijn, L.P. (1981) Climacteric symptoms according to body weight in women of different socioeconomic groups. *Maturitas*, vol. 3, pp. 279-87.
Campbell, S. (1976) *Management of Menopause and Postmenopausal Years*. MTP Press, Lancaster.
Campbell, S. and Whitehead, M. (1977) Oestrogen therapy and the menopausal syndrome. *Clinics in Obstetrics and Gynaecology*, vol. 4, pp. 31-47.
Cattell, R.B. (1966) The scree test for the number of factors. *Multivariate Behavioural Research*, vol. 1, pp. 245-53.
Chakravarti, S., Collins, W., Newton, J., Oram, D. and Studd, J. (1977) Endocrine changes and symptomatology after oophorectomy in premenopausal women. *British Journal of Obstetrics and Gynaecology*, vol. 84, pp. 769-75.
Chakravarti, W., Collins, W., Thom, M. and Studd, J. (1979) The relation between plasma hormone profiles, symptoms and response to

oestrogen treatment in women approaching the menopause. *British Medical Journal*, vol. 1, pp. 983-5.
Christenson, C. and Gagnon, J. (1965) Sexual behaviour in a group of older women. *Journal of Gerontology*, vol. 20, pp. 351-6.
Clark, A. and Wallin, P. (1965) Women's sexual responsiveness and the duration and quality of their marriages. *American Journal of Sociology*, vol. 71, pp. 187-96.
Cobb, S. (1976) Social support as a moderator of life stress. *Psychosomatic Medicine*, vol. 38, pp. 300-11.
Cohen, J. (1968) Multiple regression as a general data-analytic system. *Psychological Bulletin*, vol. 70, pp. 426-43.
Cooke, D.J. and Greene, J.G. (1981) Types of life events in relation to symptoms at the climacteric. *Journal of Psychosomatic Research*, vol. 25, pp. 5-11.
Coope, J., Thomson, J.M. and Poller, L. (1975) Effects of natural oestrogen replacement therapy on menopausal symptoms and blood clotting. *British Medical Journal*, vol. 4, pp. 139-43.
Coppen, A., Eccleston, E. and Peet, M. (1973) Total and free tryptophan concentration in the plasma of depressive patients. *The Lancet*, vol. 2, pp. 60-3.
Coppen, A. and Wood, K. (1978) Tryptophan and depressive illness. *Psychological Medicine*, vol. 8, pp. 49-57.
Council of the Medical Women's Federation (1933) An investigation of the menopause in one thousand women. *The Lancet*, vol. 1, pp. 106-8.
Crawford, M. and Hooper, D. (1973) Menopause, ageing and family. *Social Science and Medicine*, vol. 7, pp. 469-82.
Dartington, R.B. (1968) Multiple regression in psychological research and practice. *Psychological Bulletin*, vol. 69, pp. 161-82.
Davis, D.L. (1982) Women's status and experience of the menopause in a Newfoundland fishing village. *Maturitas*, vol. 4, pp. 207-16.
Davis, D.L. (1983) *Blood and Nerves: An Ethnographic Focus on Menopause*. Memorial University of Newfoundland, St John's.
Dege, K. and Gretzinger, J. (1982) Attitudes of families toward menopause, in A. Voda, M. Dinnerstein and S. O'Donnell (eds.), *Changing Perspectives on Menopause*. University of Texas Press, Austin.
Dennerstein, L., Burrows, G.D., Hyman, G. and Sharpe, K. (1979) Hormone therapy and affect. *Maturitas*, vol. 1, pp. 247-59.
Dennerstein, L., Burrows, G.D., Hyman, G. and Wood, C. (1978) Menopausal hot flushes — double blind comparison of ethinyloestradiol and norgestal. *British Journal of Obstetrics and Gynaecology*, vol. 85, pp. 852-6.

Dennerstein, L., Burrows, G., Wood, C. and Hyman, G. (1980) Hormones and sexuality: Effect of oestrogen and progestogen. *Obstetrics and Gynecology*, vol. 56, pp. 316-22.

Dennerstein, L., Wood, C. and Burrows, G. (1977) Sexual response following hysterectomy and oophorectomy. *Obstetrics and Gynecology*, vol. 49, pp. 92-6.

Dennerstein, L., Wood, C., Hudson, B. and Burrows, G. (1978) Clinical features and plasma hormone levels after surgical menopause. *Australian and New Zealand Journal of Obstetrics and Gynaecology*, vol. 18, pp. 202-5.

Dodds, D., Potgieter, C. and Turner, P. (1961) The physical and emotional results of hysterectomy: A review of 162 cases. *South African Medical Journal*, vol. 35, pp. 53-4.

Dohrenwend, B.S. and Dohrenwend, B.P. (1974) *Stressful Life Events: Their Nature and Effects*. Wiley, New York.

Dohrenwend, B.S. and Dohrenwend, B.P. (1981) *Life Stress and Illness*. Neale Watson, New York.

Donovan, J.C. (1951) Menopausal syndrome: A study of case histories. *American Journal of Obstetrics and Gynecology*, vol. 62, pp. 1281-91.

Dow, M., Hart, D. and Forrest, C. (1983) Hormonal treatments of sexual unresponsiveness in post-menopausal women: A comparative study. *British Journal of Obstetrics and Gynaecology*, vol. 90, pp. 361-6.

Dowtry, N., Maoz, B., Antonovsky, A. and Wijsenbeek, H. (1970) Climacterium in three cultural contexts. *Tropical Geographical Medicine*, vol. 22, pp. 77-86.

Dreyfus, G.L. (1907) *Die Melancholie*. Fischer, Jena.

Durst, N. and Maoz, B. (1979) Changes in psychological well-being during post-menopause as a result of estrogen therapy. *Maturitas*, vol. 1, pp. 301-5.

Eisner, H. and Kelly, L. (1980) Attitude of women toward the menopause. Paper presented at Gerontological Society Meeting, San Diego, California.

Eysenck, H.J. (1953) The logical basis of factor analysis. *American Psychologist*, vol. 8, pp. 105-14.

Eysenck, H.J. (1970) The classification of depressive illness. *British Journal of Psychiatry*, vol. 117, pp. 241-50.

Fedor-Freybergh, P. (1977) The influence of oestrogens on the wellbeing and mental performance in climacteric and postmenopausal women. *Acta Obstetrica Gynecologia Scandinavica*, suppl. 64, pp. 5-88.

Fessler, L. (1950) The psychopathology of climacteric depression. *Psychoanalytic Quarterly*, vol. 19, pp. 28-35.

Finlay-Jones, R. and Brown, G.W. (1981) Types of stressful life events and

the onset of anxiety and depressive disorders. *Psychological Medicine*, vol. 11, pp. 803-15.
Flint, R. (1975) The menopause: Reward or punishment. *Psychosomatics*, vol. 16, pp. 161-3.
Flint, M.P. (1979) Transcultural influences in perimenopause, in A. Haspels and H. Musaph (eds.), *Psychosomatics in Peri-Menopause*. MTP Press, Lancaster.
Flint, M. and Garcia, M. (1979) Culture and the climacteric. *Journal of Biosocial Science*, suppl. 6, pp. 197-215.
Freeman, H.E., Levine, S. and Reeder, L.G. (1972) *Handbook of Medical Sociology*. Prentice-Hall, New Jersey.
Frere, G. (1971) Mean age at menopause and menarche in South Africa. *South African Journal of Medical Science*, vol. 36, pp. 21-4.
Friedman, A., Cowitz, B., Cohen, H. and Granick, S. (1963) Syndromes and themes of psychotic depression. *Archives of General Psychiatry*, vol. 9, pp. 504-9.
Garde, K. and Lunde, I. (1980a) Female sexual behaviour. A study in a random sample of 40-year old women. *Maturitas*, vol. 2, pp. 225-40.
Garde, K. and Lunde, I. (1980b) Social background and social status: Influence on female sexual behaviour. A random sample study of 40-year old Danish women. *Maturitas*, vol. 2, pp. 241-6.
George, G.W.C., Utian, W.H., Beaumont, P.J.V. and Bearwood, C.J. (1973) Effects of exogenous oestrogen on minor psychiatric symptoms in postmenopausal women. *South African Medical Journal*, vol. 47, pp. 2387-8.
Gerdes, L., Sonnendecker, E. and Polakow, E. (1982) Psychological changes effected by estrogen-progestogen and clonidine treatment in climacteric women. *American Journal of Obstetrics and Gynecology*, vol. 142, pp. 98-104.
Ginsberg, S. (1976) Women, work and conflict, in N. Fonda and P. Moss (eds.), *Mothers in Employment*. Brunel University.
Goldberg, D. (1972) *The Detection of Psychiatric Illness by Questionnaire*. Oxford University Press, London.
Goldberg, D. and Huxley, P. (1980) *Mental Illness in the Community*. Tavistock Publications, London.
Gould, R. (1978) *Transformations*. Simon and Schuster, New York.
Gray, R.H. (1976) The menopause — epidemiological and demographic considerations, in R.J. Beard (ed.), *Menopause – Guide to Current Research and Practice*. MTP Press, Lancaster.
Greenblatt, R.B., Barfield, W., Garner, J., Calk, G. and Harrod, J. (1950) Evaluations of an oestrogen, androgen, oestrogen-androgen combination, and a placebo in the treatment of the menopause. *Journal of*

Clinical Endocrinology, vol. 10, pp. 1547-58.
Greenblatt, R., Cameron, N. and Karpas, A. (1980) The menopausal syndrome: Hormone replacement therapy, in B.A. Eskin (ed.), *The Menopause: Comprehensive Management*. Masson Publishers Inc., New York.
Greene, J.G. (1976) A factor analytic study of climacteric symptoms. *Journal of Psychosomatic Research*, vol. 20, pp. 425-30.
Greene, J.G. (1982) Psychosocial factors in women during the climacteric: A community study, in C.J. Main (ed.), *Clinical Psychology and Medicine: A Behavioural Perspective*. Plenum Publishing Co., New York.
Greene, J.G. (1983) Bereavement and social support at the climacteric. *Maturitas*, vol. 5, pp. 115-24.
Greene, J.G. and Cooke, D.J. (1980) Life stress and symptoms at the climacteric. *British Journal of Psychiatry*, vol. 136, pp. 486-91.
Greenhill, M.H. (1946) A psychosomatic evaluation of the psychiatric and endocrinological factors in the menopause. *Southern Medical Journal Nashville*, vol. 39, pp. 786-93.
Griffen, J. (1977) A crosscultural investigation of behavioural changes at menopause. *The Social Science Journal*, vol. 14, pp. 49-55.
Griffen, J. (1982) Cultural models for coping with the menopause, in A. Voda, M. Dinnerstein and S. O'Donnell (eds.), *Changing Perspectives on Menopause*. University of Texas Press, Austin.
Gunderson, E.K. and Rahe, R.H. (1974) *Life Stress and Illness*. Charles C. Thomas, Springfield.
Hagnell, O. (1966) *A Prospective Study of the Incidence of Mental Disorder*. Munksgaard, Copenhagen.
Hallstrom, T. (1973) *Mental Disorder and Sexuality in the Climacteric*. Scandinavian University Books, Stockholm.
Hallstrom, T. (1977) Sexuality in the climacteric. *Clinics in Obstetrics and Gynaecology*, vol. 4, pp. 227-39.
Hamilton, M. (1959) The assessment of anxiety states by rating. *British Journal of Medical Psychology*, vol. 32, pp. 50-5.
Hamilton, M. (1960) A rating scale for depression. *Journal of Neurology, Neurosurgery and Psychiatry*, vol. 23, pp. 56-62.
Hamilton, M. (1974) *Methodology of Clinical Research*. Churchill Livingstone, Edinburgh.
Haspels, A.A. and Keep, van P.A. (1979) Endocrinology and management of the peri-menopause, in A.A. Haspels and H. Musaph (eds.), *Psychosomatics in Peri-menopause*. MTP Press, Lancaster.
Haspels, A.A. and Musaph, H. (1979) *Psychosomatics in Peri-Menopause*. MTP Press, Lancaster.

Hawkinson, L.F. (1938) The menopausal syndrome. One thousand consecutive patients treated with estrogen. *Journal of the American Medical Association*, vol. 111, pp. 390-3.

Henderson, D.K. and Gillespie, R.D. (1932) *A Textbook of Psychiatry for Students and Practitioners*. Oxford University Press, New York.

Henderson, S. (1981) Social relationships, adversity and neurosis: An analysis of prospective observations. *British Journal of Psychiatry*, vol. 138, pp. 391-8.

Henderson, S., Byrne, D.G. and Duncan-Jones, P. (1981) *Neuroses and the Social Environment*. Academic Press, Sydney.

Herrman, W., McDonald, R. and Bozak, M. (1978) The effects of hormones on human behaviour as measured by psychological tests. *Progress in Neuro-Psychopharmacology*, vol. 2, pp. 469-78.

Holmes, T.H. and Rahe, R.H. (1967) The social readjustment rating scale. *Journal of Psychosomatic Research*, vol. 11, pp. 213-8.

Holte, A. and Mikkelsen, A. (1982) Menstrual coping style social background and climacteric symptoms. *Psychiatry and Social Science*, vol. 2, pp. 41-5.

Huffman, J.W. (1950) The effect of gynecologic surgey on sexual reactions. *American Journal of Obstetrics and Gynecology*, vol. 59, pp. 915-7.

Hunter, D., Akande, O., Carr, P. and Stallworthy, J. (1973) The clinical and endocrinological effect of oestradiol implants at the time of hysterectomy and bilateral salpingo-oophorectomy. *British Journal of Obstetrics and Gynaecology*, vol. 80, pp. 827-33.

Hutton, J., Murray, M., Jacobs, H. and James, V. (1978) Relation between plasma oestrone and oestradiol and climacteric symptoms. *The Lancet*, vol. 1, pp. 678-81.

Ikeda, T., Ueda, T., Kamatsuki, S., Arima, M., Mihara, K., Mori, I., Takenaka, S. and Ogawa, N. (1978) Psychosomatic aspects of the effect of conjugated estrogens in patients with postoperative ovarian deficiency syndrome. *Maturitas*, vol. 1, pp. 113-9.

Indira, S.N. and Murthy, V.N. (1980a) Nature of psychiatric disturbance in menopausal women. *Indian Journal of Clinical Psychology*, vol. 7, pp. 7-11.

Indira, S.N. and Murthy, V.N. (1980b) A factor analytic study of menopausal symptoms in middle aged women. *Indian Journal of Clinical Psychology*, vol. 7, pp. 125-8.

International Health Foundation (1969) *A Study of the Attitudes of Women in Belgium, France, Great Britain, Italy and West Germany*. IHF, Brussels.

International Health Foundation (1975) *The Mature Women: A First*

Analysis of a Psychosocial Study of Chronological and Menstrual Ageing . IHF, Geneva.

International Health Foundation (1977) *La Menopause: Etude effectuée en Belgique auprès de 922 femmes entre 45 et 55 ans*. IHF, Geneva.

Jarvinen, P.A., Kokkenen, J. and Rhyanen, P. (1971) Oestriol succinate in the treatment of climacteric women: A double-blind trial. *Acta Obstetrica Gynecologia Scandinavica*, vol. 50, suppl. 9.

Jaszmann, L., Van Lith, N. and Zaat, J. (1969a) The age at menopause in the Netherlands. *International Journal of Fertility*, vol. 14, pp. 106-17.

Jaszmann, L., Van Lith, N. and Zaat, J. (1969b) The perimenopausal symptoms: The statistical analysis of a survey. *Medical Gynaecology and Sociology*, vol. 4, pp. 268-77.

Kantor, H., Michael, C., Shore, H. and Ludvigson, H. (1968) Administration of estrogens to older women, a psychometric evaluation. *American Journal of Obstetrics and Gynecology*, vol. 101, pp. 658-61.

Kantor, H., Milton, L. and Ernst, M. (1978) Comparative psychologic effects of estrogen administration on institutional and noninstitutional elderly women. *Journal of the American Geriatrics Society*, vol. 36, pp. 9-16.

Kaufert, P. (1982) Anthropology and the menopause: The development of a theoretical framework. *Maturitas*, vol. 4, pp. 181-93.

Kaufert, P. and Syrotuik, J. (1981) Symptom reporting at the menopause. *Social Science and Medicine*, vol. 15, pp. 173-84.

Kearns, B.J. (1982) Perceptions of menopause by Papago women, in A. Voda, M. Dinnerstein and S. O'Donnell (eds.), *Changing Perspectives on Menopause*. University of Texas Press, Austin.

Keep, P.A. van (1975) Psycho-sociology of menopause and postmenopause. *Frontiers in Hormone Research*, vol. 3, pp. 32-9.

Keep, P.A. van (1979) Editorial note. *Maturitas*, vol. 1, p. 227.

Keep, P.A. van and Gregory, A. (1977) Sexual relations in the ageing female, in J. Money and H. Musaph (eds.), *Handbook of Sexology*. Elsevier, North Holland Biomedical Press.

Keep, P.A. van and Kellerhals, J. (1973) The ageing women. *Frontiers in Hormone Research*, vol. 2, pp. 160-73.

Keep, P.A. van and Kellerhals, J. (1974) The impact of socio-cultural factors on symptom formation: Some results of a study on ageing women in Switzerland. *Psychotherapy and Psychosomatics*, vol. 23, pp. 251-63.

Keep, P.A. van and Kellerhals, J. (1975) The ageing woman: About the influence of some social and cultural factors on the change in attitude and behaviour that occur during and after the menopause. *Acta*

Obstetrica Gynecologia Scandinavica, suppl. 51, pp. 17-27.
Keep, P.A. van, Serr, D.M. and Greenblatt, R.B. (1979) *Female and Male Climacteric: Current Opinion*. MTP Press, Lancaster.
Kellner, R. and Sheffield, B. (1973) A self-rating scale of distress. *Psychological Medicine*, vol. 5, pp. 88-100.
Kendell, R.E. and Gourlay, J. (1970) The clinical distinction between psychotic and neurotic depression. *British Journal of Psychiatry*, vol. 117, pp. 257-66.
Kerr, M.D. (1976) Psychological changes following hormonal therapy, in S. Campbell (ed.), *The Management of the Menopause and Post-Menopausal Years*. MTP Press, Lancaster.
Kiloh, L., Andrews, G., Neilson, M. and Bianchi, G. (1972) The relationship of the syndromes called endogenous and neurotic depression. *British Journal of Psychiatry*, vol. 121, pp. 183-96.
Kiloh, L. and Garside, R. (1963) The independence of neurotic and endogenous depression. *British Journal of Psychiatry*, vol. 109, pp. 451-63.
Kinsey, A.C., Pomeroy, W., Martin, C. and Gebhard, P. (1953) *Sexual Behaviour in the Human Female*. Saunders, Philadelphia.
Kopera, H. (1973) Estrogens and psychic functions. *Frontiers in Hormone Research*, vol. 2, pp. 118-33.
Krystal, S. and Chiriboga, D. (1979) The empty nest process in mid-life man and women. *Maturitas*, vol. 1, pp. 215-22.
Kupperman, H.S., Blatt, M.G., Wiesbader, H. and Filler, W. (1953) Comparative clinical evaluation of estrogenic preparations by the menopausal and amenorrheal indices. *Journal of Clinical Endocrinology*, vol. 13, pp. 688-703.
Kupperman, H.S., Wetchler, B.B. and Blatt, M.G. (1959) Contemporary therapy of the menopausal syndrome. *Journal of the American Medical Association*, vol. 171, pp. 1627-37.
Lauritzen, C. (1973) The management of the pre-menopausal and the post-menopausal patient. *Frontiers in Hormone Research*, vol. 2, pp. 2-21.
Lauritzen, C. and Keep, P.A. van (1978) Proven beneficial effects of estrogen substitution in the post-menopause: A review. *Frontiers in Hormone Research*, vol. 5, pp. 1-25.
Lawley, D.N. and Maxwell, A.E. (1963) *Factor Analysis as a Statistical Method*. Butterworths, London.
Lennon, M.C. (1980) Psychological reactions to menopause: A sociological study. *Dissertation Abstracts International*, vol. 41, p. 4182.
Levinson, D.J. (1978) *The Seasons of Man's Life*. Knopf Inc., New York.
Levit, L. (1963) *Anxiety and the Menopause: A Study of Normal Women*.

Unpublished doctoral dissertation, University of Chicago.
Lewis, A.J. (1934) Melancholia: A clinical survey of depressive states. *Journal of Mental Science*, vol. 80, pp. 277-378.
Lincoln, N.L. (1980) Women's attitudes toward menopause as related to self-esteem. *Dissertation Abstracts International*, vol. 41, p. 3630.
Lowenthal, M.F. and Chiriboga, D. (1972) Transitions to the empty nest: Crisis, challenge or relief. *Archives of General Psychiatry*, vol. 26, pp. 8-14.
Lozman, H., Barlow, A.L. and Levitt, D.G. (1971) Piperazine oestrone sulphate and conjugated oestrogen equine in the treatment of the menopausal syndrome. *Southern Medical Journal*, vol. 64, pp. 1143-9.
MacMahon, B. and Worcester, J. (1966) Age at menopause: United States, 1960-62. *U.S. Vital and Health Statistics*, vol. 11, pp. 11-20.
Maoz, B., Antonovsky, A., Apter, A., Wijsenbeek, H. and Datan, N. (1977) The perception of menopause in five ethnic groups in Israel. *Acta Obstetrica Gynecologia Scandinavica*, suppl. 65, pp. 69-76.
Maoz, B., Antonovsky, A., Apter, A., Datan, N., Hochberg, J. and Salomon, Y. (1978) The effect of outside work on the menopausal woman. *Maturitas*, vol. 1, pp. 43-53.
Maoz, B., Dowtry, N., Antonovsky, A. and Wijsenbeek, H. (1970) Female attitudes to menopause. *Social Psychiatry*, vol. 5, pp. 35-40.
Maoz, B. and Durst, N. (1980) The effects of oestrogen on the sex life of post-menopausal women. *Maturitas*, vol. 2, pp. 327-36.
McKinlay, S. and Jefferys, M. (1974) The menopausal syndrome. *British Journal of Preventative and Social Medicine*, vol. 28, pp. 108-15.
McKinlay, S. Jefferys, M. and Thompson, B. (1972) An investigation of the age at menopause. *Journal of Biosocial Science*, vol. 4, pp. 161-73.
Martin, P.L., Burnier, A.M., Segre, E. and Huix, F.J. (1971) Graded sequential therapy in the menopause: A double blind trial. *American Journal of Obstetrics and Gynecology*, vol. 111, pp. 178-86.
Masters, W.H. and Johnson, V.E. (1966) *Human Sexual Response*. Little, Brown & Co., Boston.
Mayer-Gross, W., Slater, E. and Roth, M. (1955) *Clinical Psychiatry*. Williams and Wilkins, Baltimore.
Michael, C.M., Kantor, H.J. and Shore, H. (1970) Further psychometric evaluation of older women: The effect of estrogen administration. *Journal of Gerontology*, vol. 25, pp. 337-41.
Mikkelsen, A. and Holte, A. (1982) A factor-analytic study of climacteric symptoms. *Psychiatry and Social Science*, vol. 2, pp. 35-9.
Miller, P. and Ingham, J.G. (1976) Friends, confidants and symptoms. *Social Psychiatry*, vol. 11, pp. 51-8.
Miller, P., Ingham, J.G. and Davidson, S. (1976) Life events, symptoms

and social support. *Journal of Psychosomatic Research*, vol. 20, pp. 515-22.

Moore, B. (1981) Climacteric symptoms in an African community. *Maturitas*, vol. 3, pp. 25-9.

Moore, B., Gustafson, R. and Studd, J. (1975) Experience of a National Health Service menopause clinic. *Current Medical Research and Opinion*, suppl. 3, pp. 42-55.

Morris, J.N. (1975) *The Uses of Epidemiology*. Churchill Livingstone, Edinburgh.

Mulley, G. and Mitchell, J. (1976) Menopausal flushing: Does oestrogen therapy make sense? *The Lancet*, vol. 1, pp. 1397-9.

Munro, A. (1969) Psychiatric illness in gynaecological out patients — A preliminary study. *British Journal of Psychiatry*, vol. 115, pp. 807-9.

Neugarten, B.L. (1968) *Middle Age and Ageing*. University of Chicago Press, Chicago.

Neugarten, B.L. (1979) Time, age and the life cycle. *American Journal of Psychiatry*, vol. 136, pp. 887-94.

Neugarten, B.L. and Datan, N. (1974) The middle years, in S. Arieti (ed.), *American Handbook of Psychiatry*. Basic Books, New York.

Neugarten, B.L. and Kraines, R. (1965) Menopausal symptoms in women of various ages. *Psychosomatic Medicine*, vol. 27, pp. 266-73.

Neugarten, B.L., Wood, V., Kraines, R. and Loomis, B. (1963) Women's attitudes toward the menopause. *Vita Humana*, vol. 6, pp. 140-51.

Nordin, B.E., Jones, M.M., Crilly, R.G., Marshall, D.H. and Brooke, R. (1980) A placebo-controlled trial of ethinyloestradiol and norethisterone in climacteric women. *Maturitas*, vol. 2, pp. 247-51.

Notman, M. (1979) Midlife concerns of women: Implications of the menopause. *American Journal of Psychiatry*, vol. 136, pp. 1270-4.

Oram, D. and Chakravarti, S. (1975) The pathology of the menopause and climacteric. *Current Medical Reseach and Opinion*, suppl. 3, pp. 11-9.

Osofsky, H. and Seidenberg, R. (1970) Is female menopausal depression inevitable? *Obstetrics and Gynecology*, vol. 36, pp. 613-5.

Parkes, C.M. (1971) Psycho-social transitions: A field for study. *Social Science and Medicine*, vol. 5, pp. 101-15.

Parry, G., Shapiro, D.A. and Davies, L. (1981) Reliability of life-event ratings: An independent replication. *British Journal of Social and Clinical Psychology*, vol. 20, pp. 133-4.

Paterson, M.E.L. (1982) A randomised, double-blind cross-over study into the effect of sequential mestranol and norethisterone on climacteric symptoms and biochemical parameters. *Maturitas*, vol. 4, pp. 83-94.

Patterson, R. and Craig, J. (1963) Misconceptions concerning the psychological effects of hysterectomy. *American Journal of Obstetrics and Gynecology*, vol. 85, pp. 104-11.

Paykel, E.S., Emms, E.M., Fletcher, J. and Rassaby, E. (1980) Life events and social support in puerperal depression. *British Journal of Psychiatry*, vol. 136, pp. 339-46.

Paykel, E.S., McGuiness, B. and Gomez, J. (1976) An Anglo-American comparison of the scaling of life events. *British Journal of Medical Psychology*, vol. 49, pp. 237-47.

Paykel, E.S., Myers, J.K., Dienelt, M.N., Klerman, G.L., Lindethal, J. and Pepper, M. (1969) Life events and depression: A controlled study. *Archives of General Psychiatry*, vol. 21, pp. 753-60.

Paykel, E.S., Prusoff, B.A. and Myers, J.K. (1975) Suicide attempt and recent life events. *Archives of General Psychiatry*, vol. 32, pp. 327-33.

Paykel, E.S., Prusoff, B.A. and Uhlenhuth, E.H. (1971) Scaling of life events. *Archives of General Psychiatry*, vol. 25, pp. 340-7.

Peet, M., Moody, J., Worrall, E., Walker, P. and Naylor, G. (1976) Plasma tryptophan concentration in depressive illness and mania. *British Journal of Psychiatry*, vol. 128, pp. 255-8.

Perlmutter, E. (1981) Women's views of menopause: An experimental approach. *Dissertation Abstracts International*, vol. 42, p. 2076.

Perlmutter, E. and Bart, P.B. (1982) Changing views of "the change": A critical review and suggestions for an attributional approach, in A. Voda, M. Dinnerstein and S. O'Donnell (eds.), *Changing Perspectives on Menopause*. University of Texas Press, Austin.

Pfeiffer, E. and Davis, G. (1972) Determinants of sexual behaviour in middle and old age. *Journal of the American Geriatrics Association*, vol. 20, pp. 151-8.

Pfeiffer, E., Verwoerdt, A. and Davis, G. (1972) Sexual behaviour in middle life. *American Journal of Psychiatry*, vol. 128, pp. 1262-7.

Polit, D. and Larocco, S. (1980) Social and psychological correlates of menopausal symptoms. *Psychosomatic Medicine*, vol. 42, pp. 335-45.

Pratt, J.P. and Thomas, W.L. (1937) The endocrine treatment of menopausal phenomenon. *Journal of the American Medical Association*, vol. 109, pp. 1875-80.

Prill, H.J. (1966) Die Beziehung von Erkrankungen und socialpsychologischen Fakten zum Klimacterium. *Medizinische Klinik*, vol. 61, pp. 325-8.

Prill, H.J. (1977) A study of the socio-medical relationships at the climacteric in 2232 women. *Current Medical Research and Opinion*, suppl. 3, pp. 46-51.

Prudo, R., Brown, G.W., Harris, T. and Dowland, J. (1981) Psychiatric disorder in a rural and an urban population: 2. Sensitivity to loss. *Psychological Medicine*, vol. 11, pp. 601-16.

Rauramo, L., Lagerspetz, L., Engblom, P. and Punnonen, R. (1975) The effect of castration and peroral estrogen therapy on some psychological functions. *Frontiers in Hormone Research*, vol. 3, pp. 94-104.

Richards, D.H. (1973) A post-hysterectomy syndrome. *The Lancet*, vol. 2, pp. 430-3.

Rosenthal, S. (1968) The involutional depressive syndrome. *American Journal of Psychiatry*, vol. 124 (suppl.), pp. 21-35.

Rosenthal, S. and Gudeman, J. (1967) The endogenous depressive pattern: An empirical investigation. *Archives of General Psychiatry*, vol. 113, pp. 85-9.

Rosenthal, S. and Klerman, G. (1966) Content and consistency in the endogenous depressive pattern. *British Journal of Psychiatry*, vol. 112, pp. 471-84.

Rossi, A.A. (1980) Life-span theories and women's lives. *Signs: Journal of Women in Society and Culture*, vol. 6, pp. 4-32.

Roth, M. (1959) The phenomenology of depressive states. *Canadian Psychiatric Association Journal*, vol. 4 (suppl.), pp. 32-54.

Roth, M., Gurney, C., Garside, R. and Kerr, T. (1972) Studies in the classification of affective disorders: The relationship between anxiety states and depressive illness. *British Journal of Psychiatry*, vol. 121, pp. 147-61.

Rybo, G. and Westerberg, H. (1971) Symptoms in the postmenopause: A population study. *Acta Obstetrica Gynecologia Scandinavica*, suppl. 9, p. 25.

Sainsbury, P. (1960) Psychosomatic disorders and neurosis in outpatients attending a general hospital. *Journal of Psychosomatic Research*, vol. 4, pp. 261-73.

Schachter, S. (1964) The interaction of cognitive and physiological determinants of emotional states, in L. Berkowitz (ed.), *Advances in Experimental Social Psychology*. Academic Press, New York.

Schiff, I., Regestein, Q., Tulchinsky, D. and Ryan, K. (1979) Effects of estrogens on sleep and psychological state of hypogonadal women. *Journal of the American Medical Association*, vol. 242, pp. 2405-7.

Schneider, M. and Brotherton, P. (1979) Physiological, psychological and situational stresses in depression during the climacteric. *Maturitas*, vol. 1, pp. 153-8.

Schneider, M., Brotherton, P. and Hailes, J. (1977) The effect of exogenous oestrogens on depression in menopausal women. *Medical Journal of Australia*, vol. 2, pp. 162-3.

Severne, L. (1977) *Le Deuxième Age Adulte: Un portrait statistique de la femme belge autour de la cinquantaine.* International Health Foundation, Geneva.

Severne, L. (1979) Psycho-social aspects of the menopause, in A. Haspels and H. Musaph (eds.), *Psychosomatics in Peri-Menopause.* MTP Press, Lancaster.

Severne, L. (1982) Psychosocial aspects of the menopause, in A. Voda, M. Dinnerstein and S. O'Donnell (eds.), *Changing Perspectives on Menopause.* University of Texas Press, Austin.

Sevringhaus, E.L. (1935) The relief of menopause symptoms by estrogenic preparations. *Journal of the American Medical Association*, vol. 104, pp. 624-6.

Shapiro, M.B. (1979) The Social Origins of Depression by G.W. Brown and T. Harris: Its methodological philosophy *Behavour Research and Therapy*, vol. 17, pp. 597-603.

Sharma, V. and Saxena, M. (1981) Climacteric symptoms: A Study in the Indian context. *Maturitas*, vol. 3, pp. 11-20.

Sheehy, G. (1976) *Passages.* Dutton and Co., New York.

Sherman, B., West, J. and Korenman, S. (1976) The menopausal transition: Analysis of LH, FSH, estradiol and progesterone concentrations during menstrual cycles of older women. *Journal of Clinical Endocrinology and Metabolism*, vol. 42, pp. 629-36.

Sonnendecker, E. and Polakow, E. (1980) A comparison of oestrogen-progesteron with clonidine in the climacteric syndrome. *South African Medical Journal*, vol. 58, pp. 753-6.

Spanier, G.B. (1976) Measuring dyadic adjustment: New scales for assessing the quality of marriage and similar dyads. *Journal of Marriage and the Family*, vol. 38, pp. 15-28.

Stern, K. and Prados, M. (1946) Personality studies in menopausal women. *American Journal of Psychiatry*, vol. 103, pp. 358-68.

Stone, S., Mickal, A., Rye, P. and Phillip, H. (1975) Postmenopausal symptomatology, maturation index, and plasma estrogen levels. *Obstetrics and Gynecology*, vol. 45, pp. 625-7.

Strickler, R., Borth, R., Cecutti, A., Cookson, B., Harper, J., Potvin, P., Sorbara, V. and Woolever, C. (1977) The role of oestrogen replacement in the climacteric syndrome. *Psychological Medicine*, vol. 7, pp. 631-9.

Studd, J., Chakravarti, S. and Orman, D. (1975) Practical aspects of hormone replacement therapy. *Current Medical Research and Opinion*, suppl. 3, pp. 56-65.

Studd, J., Chakravarti, S. and Oram, D. (1977a) The climacteric *Clinics in Obstetrics and Gynaecology*, vol. 4, no. 1, pp. 3-29.

Studd, J., Collins, W., Chakravarti, S., Newton, J., Oram, D. and Parsons, A. (1977b) Oestradiol and testosterone implants in the treatment of psychosexual problems in post-menopausal women. *British Journal of Obstetrics and Gynaecology*, vol. 84, pp. 314-5.

Studd, J. and Parsons, A. (1977) Sexual dysfunction: The climacteric. *British Journal of Sexual Medicine*, vol. 4, pp. 11-2.

Tait, A.C., Harper, J. and McClatchey, W.T. (1957) Initial psychiatric illness in involutional women. *Journal of Mental Science*, vol. 103, pp. 132-45.

Tanner, J.M. (1962) *Growth at Adolescence*. Blackwell, Oxford.

Tennant, C. and Andrews, G. (1978) The pathogenic quality of life events in neurotic impairment. *Archives of General Psychiatry*, vol. 35, pp. 859-63.

Tennant, C. and Bebbington, P. (1978) The social causation of depression: A critique of the work of Brown and his colleagues. *Psychological Medicine*, vol. 8, pp. 565-75.

Thompson, B., Hart, S. and Durno, D. (1973) Menopausal age and symptomatology in general practice. *Journal of Biosocial Science*, vol. 5, pp. 71-82.

Thomson, J. and Oswald, I. (1977) Effect of oestrogen on the sleep, mood and anxiety of menopausal women. *British Medical Journal*, vol. 2, pp. 1317-9.

Townsend, P., Whitehead, M., McQueen, J., Minardi, J. and Campbell, S. (1980) Double-blind studies of the effects of natural estrogens on postmenopausal women: A follow up report, in N. Pasetto, R. Paoletti and J. Ambrus (eds.), *The Menopause and Postmenopause*. MTP Press, Lancaster.

Tucket, D.A. (1976) *An Introduction to Medical Sociology*. Tavistock Publications, London.

Uphold, C. and Susman, E. (1981) Self-reported climacteric symptoms as a function of the relationship between marital adjustment and child rearing stage. *Nursing Research*, vol. 30, pp. 84-8.

Utian, W.H. (1972a) The true clinical features of the post-menopause and oophorectomy and their response to oestrogen therapy. *South African Medical Journal*, vol. 46, pp. 732-7.

Utian, W.H. (1972b) The mental tonic effect of oestrogen administered to oophorectomised females. *South African Medical Journal*, vol. 46, pp. 1079-82.

Utian, W.H. (1975) Effect of hysterectomy, oophorectomy and estrogen therapy on libido. *International Journal of Gynaecology and Obstetrics*, vol. 13, pp. 97-100.

Utian, W.H. (1980) *Menopause in Modern Perspective: A Guide to Clinical Practice*. Appleton Century Crofts, New York.

Utian, W.H. and Serr, D. (1976) Report on workshop: The climacteric syndrome, in P.A. van Keep, R.B. Greenblatt and M. Albeaux-Fernet (eds.), *Consensus on Menopause Research*. MTP Press, Lancaster.

Vaillant, G.E. (1977) *Adaptation to Life*. Little, Brown & Co., Boston.

Vanhulle, G. and Demol, R. (1976) A double-blind study into the influence of estriol on a number of psychological tests in postmenopausal women, in P.A. van Keep, R.B. Greenblatt and M. Albeaux-Fernet (eds.), *Consensus on Menopause Research*. MTP Press, Lancaster.

Voda, A., Dinnerstein, M. and O'Donnell, S. (1982) *Changing Perspectives on Menopause*, University of Texas Press, Austin.

Warr, P. (1983) Work, jobs and unemployment. *Bulletin of the British Psychological Society*, vol. 36, pp. 305-11.

Weissman, M.M. (1979) The myth of involutional melancholia. *Journal of the American Medical Association*, vol. 242, pp. 742-4.

Weissman, M.M. and Klerman, G. (1977) Sex differences and the epidemiology of depression. *Archives of General Psychiatry*, vol. 34, pp. 98-111.

Weissman, M.M. and Myers, J.K. (1978) Rates and risks of depressive symptoms in a United States urban community. *Acta Psychiatrica Scandinavica*, vol. 57, pp. 219-31.

Wenderlein, J.M. (1980) Psychotherapeutic effects of estrogen substitution during the climacteric period, in N. Pasetto, R. Paoletti and J.L. Ambrus (eds.), *The Menopause and Postmenopause*. MTP Press, Lancaster.

Wiesbader, H. and Kurzrok, R. (1938) The menopause: A consideration of the symptoms, etiology and treatment by means of estrogens. *Endocrinology*, vol. 23, pp. 32-8.

Wilbush, J. (1982) Climacteric expression and social context. *Maturitas*, vol. 4, pp. 195-205.

Williams, P., Tarnopolsky, A. and Hand, D. (1980) Case definition and case identification in psychiatric epidemiology: Review and assessment. *Psychological Medicine*, vol. 10, pp. 101-4.

Wilson, R.A. (1966) *Feminine Forever*. Mayflower-Dell, New York.

Wilson, R.A. and Wilson, T.A. (1963) The fate of the nontreated postmenopausal woman: A plea for the maintenance of adequate estrogen from puberty to the grave. *Journal of the American Geriatric Society*, vol. 11, pp. 347-53.

Wing, J., Mann, S., Leff, J. and Nixon, J. (1978) The concept of a "case" in psychiatric population surveys. *Psychological Medicine*, vol. 8, pp. 203-17.

Winokur, G. (1973) Depression in the menopause. *American Journal of Psychiatry*, vol. 130, pp. 92-3.
Wood, C. (1979) Menopausal myths. *Medical Journal of Australia*, vol. 1, pp. 496-9.
World Health Organisation (1977) *The Ninth Revision of the International Classification of Diseases*. HMSO, London.
Worsley, A., Walters, W. and Wood, E. (1977) Screening for psychological disturbance amongst gynaecology patients. *Australia and New Zealand Journal of Obstetrics and Gynaecology*, vol. 17, pp. 214-9.
Wright, A.L. (1981a) On the calculation of climacteric symptoms. *Maturitas*, vol. 3, pp. 55-63.
Wright, A.L. (1981b) Attitudes toward childbearing and menstruation among the Navajo, in M. Kay (ed.), *Anthropology of Human Birth*. F.A. Davis, Philadelphia.
Wright, A.L. (1982) Variation in Navajo menopause: Toward an explanation, in A. Voda, M. Dinnerstein and S. O'Donnell (eds.), *Changing Perspectives on Menopause*. University of Texas Press, Austin.
Wyon, J., Finner, S. and Gordon, J. (1966) Differential age at menopause in the rural Punjab, India. *Population Index*, vol. 32, p. 328.

Author Index

Adelstein, A. 96
Aksel, S 5
Amundsen, D. 3
Anastasi, A. 171
Andrews, G. 188, 190
Aylward, M. 19-22, 32

Ballinger, C.B. 27, 41, 43, 55-6, 69, 80-1, 92, 97, 103
Bancroft, J. 80
Bart, P. 102, 115, 136, 142, 150-1, 155, 157
Beaumont, P.J.V. 23

Beard, R.J. 135
Beardwood, C.J. 23
Bebbington, P. 201
Beck, A. 19, 22-3, 27, 31, 111
Belforte, L. 119
Belforte, P. 119
Blatt, M.H. 16, 174
Block, E. 2
Bodnar, S. 14
Bolding, O.T. 34
Bottiglioni, F. 84
Brand, P.4
Brooke, R. 30

Brooks-Gunn, J. 135, 146
Brotherton, P. 104, 111, 132
Brown, G.W. 187-91, 201-8, 217-8
Bungay, G. 43, 66-9, 80-1, 103, 169
Burch, P. 4
Burnier, A.M. 18
Burrows, G.D. 27

Campagnoli, C. 119-24, 129-32
Campbell, S. 19, 25-38, 88, 135
Cattell, R.B. 176
Catterill, T.B. 14
Chakravarti, S. 5, 14, 28, 33, 38, 86
Chiriboga, D. 104, 109-12, 115, 197
Christenson, C. 82
Clark, A. 83
Cobb, S. 205
Cohen, J. 192
Cooke, D.J. 43, 60-3, 69, 118-24, 129-32, 169, 183. 192, 194
Coope, J. 19, 24, 32, 63
Coppen, A. 20-1, 31-2
Craig, J. 86
Crawford, M. 102, 104, 107-8, 131, 166-7
Crilly, R.G. 30

Dartington, R.B. 192
Datan, N. 101
Davis, D.L. 148, 157-8, 170-1
Davis, G. 83
Dege, K. 136, 140, 143
De Aloysio, D. 84
Demol, R. 34
Dennerstein, L. 5, 19, 27-30, 33, 38, 86-9, 135
Diers, C. 3
Dodds, D. 86

Dohrenwend, B.P. 187
Dohrenwend, B.S. 187
Donovan, J.C. 97
Dow, M. 90
Dowtry, N. 148-9, 160
Dreyfus, G.L. 93
Durno, D. 50
Durst, N. 36, 39, 88

Eisner, H. 135-6, 139-40, 143
Eysenck, H.J. 35, 174

Fedor-Freybergh, P. 19, 25, 32, 34-5, 39, 88
Fessler, L. 97
Finlay-Jones, R. 205
Flint, R. 148, 150-1
Freeman, H.E. 116
Frere, G. 4
Friedman, A. 94

Gagnon, J. 83
Garcia, M. 148, 150
Garde, K. 85, 116, 125
Garside, R. 94
George, G.W.C. 19, 23, 31-2
Gerdes, L. 34, 36, 39
Gillespie, R.D. 93
Ginsberg, S. 216
Goldberg, D. 27, 55-6, 70
Gould, R. 102
Gourlay, J. 94
Gray, R.H. 3, 4
Greenblatt, R.B. 16, 39
Greene, J.G. 8, 43, 60-3, 69, 118-24, 129-32, 169, 175, 177-83, 192-8
Greenhill M.H. 97
Gregory, A. 91
Gretzinger, J. 136, 140, 143
Griffen, J. 146-7, 150, 213
Grossman, M. 102, 151

Gudeman, J. 94
Gunderson, E.K. 187
Gunz, F. 4

Hagnell, O. 96
Hallstrom, T. 83-5, 90, 96, 116, 125, 131
Hamilton, M. 19-21, 25-8, 32, 94, 166, 182
Harris, T. 187, 201, 205, 216
Hart, S. 50
Haspels, A.A. 13, 17, 135
Hawkinson, L.F. 15-6
Henderson, D.K. 93
Henderson, S. 187, 205
Herrmann, W. 34
Holmes, T.H. 187-9
Holte, A. 43, 65, 69, 103-6, 123, 130, 175, 180-2, 219
Hooper, D. 102, 104, 107-8, 131, 166-7
Huffman, J.W. 86
Huix, F.J. 18
Hunter, D. 5
Hutton, J. 5
Huxley, P. 56, 70
Hyman, G. 27

Ikeda, T. 19, 30-3
Indira, S.N. 41, 175, 178-82
Ingham, J.G. 205

Jarvinen, P.A. 19, 20, 31-2, 38
Jaszmann, L. 4, 43, 47-53, 57, 59, 63-4, 69-71, 113, 117-21, 130, 166, 168, 173
Jefferys, M. 43, 50-3, 63, 69-72, 116, 120, 130, 171, 191
Johnson, V.E. 83
Jones, M.M. 30

Kantor, H. 35, 36

Kaufert, P. 43, 57, 63-4, 69, 151, 166, 175, 178-82, 216
Kearns, B.J. 148, 161
Keep, P.A.van 6, 9, 13, 17, 35, 39, 43, 57-8, 69, 77, 80, 85, 91, 103-6, 116, 123-5, 130, 135, 167, 169, 171
Kellerhals, J. 6, 43, 57-8, 69, 77, 80, 85, 103-6, 116, 123-5, 130, 135, 169
Kellner, R. 175
Kelly, L. 135-6, 139-40
Kendell, R.E. 94
Kerr, M.D. 14
Kiloh, L. 94
Kinsey, A.C. 82, 88
Klerman, G. 94, 97
Kokkenen, J. 20
Kopera, H. 14, 35, 39
Kraines, R. 7, 41-6, 49, 54-5, 69, 70, 113, 137, 153, 167, 169, 173
Krystal, S. 104, 110, 112
Kuppermann, H.S. 16, 19, 20, 24, 174
Kurzrok, R. 15

Larocco, S. 121-4, 129-32
Lauritzen, C. 14, 35, 39
Lawley, D.N. 174
Lennon, M.C. 123
Levinson, D.J. 102
Levit, L. 115
Lewis, A.J. 93
Lincoln, N.L. 141
Lowenthal, M.F. 104, 109, 115, 197
Lozman, H. 22
Lunde, I. 85, 116, 125

MacMahon, B. 3, 4
McKinlay, S. 4, 43, 50-3, 56, 59,

60, 63, 65, 69-72, 116, 120, 130, 167-8, 171, 191
McPherson, C. 66
Maoz, B. 36, 39, 88, 136, 143-8, 153-4, 166
Marshall, D.H. 30
Martin, P.L. 18-21, 31-2
Masters, W.H. 83
Maxwell, A.E. 174
Mayer-Gross, W. 93
Michael, C.M. 35
Mikkelsen, A. 43, 65, 69, 103-6, 123, 130, 175, 180-2, 219
Miller, P. 205-6
Mitchell, J. 13
Moore, B. 39, 148, 152
Morra, G. 119
Morris, J.N. 116
Mulley, G. 13
Munro, A. 41
Murthy, V.N. 41, 175, 178-82
Musaph, H. 135
Myers, J.K. 96

Neugarten, B.L. 7, 42-9, 54-5, 69, 70, 101-2, 113, 136-43, 146, 153, 157, 166-9
Nordin, B.E. 19, 30, 32
Notman, M. 102

Oram, D. 14
Osofsky, H. 96
Oswald, I. 19-22, 28-9, 32-8

Parkes, C.M. 102
Parry, G. 191
Parsons, A. 80, 89
Paterson, M.E.L. 19, 29, 32, 88
Patterson, R. 86
Paykel, E.S. 187-94, 205
Peet, M. 22
Perlmutter, E. 136, 142-3

Pfeiffer, E. 83
Polakow, E. 37
Polit, D. 121-4, 129-32
Poller, L. 24
Prados, M. 97
Pratt, J.P. 16
Prill, H.J. 120-2, 129-30. 154
Prudo, R. 203

Rahe, R.H. 189-9
Rauramo, L. 33
Regestein, Q. 28
Rhyanen, P. 20
Richards, D.H. 86
Rosenthal, S. 92, 94, 97
Rossi, A.A. 102
Roth, M. 93-4
Ryan, K. 28
Rybo, G. 43, 49, 69

Sainsbury, P. 41
Saxena, M. 43, 54-5, 69-71
Schachter, S. 142
Schiff, I. 19, 28, 32, 35
Schneider, M. 30, 32, 104, 111, 132
Segre, E. 18
Seidenberg, R. 96
Serr, D. 8, 13, 100, 167, 209
Severne, L. 43, 59, 60, 64, 69, 78-9, 126-32, 141, 154-5, 173
Sevringhaus, E.L. 15
Shapiro, M.B. 190
Sharpe, K. 27
Sharma, V. 43, 54-5, 69-71
Sheehy, G. 102
Sheffield, B. 175
Sherman, B. 4
Sonnendecker, E. 37
Spanier, G.B. 113, 166
Stern, K. 97
Stone, S. 5

Strickler, R. 19, 23, 32, 34, 38
Studd, J. 4, 5, 14, 39, 80, 89-91
Susman, E. 104, 112-4, 132, 166
Syrotuik, J. 43, 57, 63-4, 69, 166, 175, 178-82

Tait, A.C. 93
Tanner, J.M. 3
Tennant, C. 188, 190, 201
Thomas, W.L. 16
Thompson, B. 4, 43, 50-2, 69, 70, 120, 171
Thomson, J. 19-22, 28-9, 32, 38
Thomson, J.M. 24
Tousijn, L.P. 119
Townsend, P. 88
Tucket, D.A. 116
Tulchinsky, D. 28

Uphold, C. 104, 112-4, 132, 166
Utian, W.H. 1, 5-8, 13, 15, 18, 19, 22-4, 32-3, 86-8, 100, 167, 209

Vaillant, G.E. 102
Vanhulle, G. 34
Van Lith, N. 47, 117

Vessay, M. 66
Voda, A. 135

Wallin, P. 83
Warr, P. 214
Weissman, M.M. 94-7
Wenderlein, J.M. 36, 39
Westerberg, H. 43, 49, 69
Whitehead, M. 19, 25-38, 88
Wiesbader, H. 15
Wilbush, J. 151, 163, 171
Williams, P. 55, 98
Willicut, H. 34
Wilson, R.A. 17
Wilson, T.A. 17
Wing, J. 55, 98
Winokur, G. 96
Wood, C. 43, 66, 68-9, 169
Wood, K. 21, 31-2
Worcester, J. 3-4
Worsley, A. 41
Wright, A.L. 148, 155-6, 159, 171
Wyon, J. 3

Zaat, J 47, 117

Subject Index

Age
    attitudes and 137-9, 143
    climacteric 4, 169
    menopausal 3-4
    symptoms and 44-7, 57-9, 66-70

Atrophic vaginitis 5, 22, 25-8, 210

Attitudes to menopause
    age and 137-9, 143
    attribution theory of 142-3
    change in 139
    cultural stability and 153-7
    cultural variation in 147-50, 153, 157
    educational level and 140-1
    European survey of 141-2
    family 140-1
    measurement of 137, 144
    psychosexual factors and 143-6
    role and status and 150-2
    social deprivation and

243

157-60
socioeconomic status and 139-41
stereotype of menopause and 141

Attribution theory 142-3

Bereavement 199, 203-4, 214-5

Causal models 206-8, 209-19

Child bearing role 102, 144, 149-52, 156, 160, 212

Child rearing role 103-15

Climacteric
    conceptual definition of 8-11
    hormones and 4
    operational definitions of 169
    ovarian failure and 4
    vulnerability 202

Climacteric symptoms
    age and 44-7, 57-9, 66-70
    assessment of 170-4, 183-5
    attitudes and 151-4, 157
    checklists of 171-3
    cultural factors and 151-7, 214-5
    cultural stability and 153-7
    departure of children and 101-15
    educational level and 116-7, 121-3
    employment and 116, 120-1, 127-31, 214, 216
    factor analysis of 174-82
    life events and 190-208
    loss of reproductive function and 111, 144, 149-52, 156, 212
    marital relations and 108, 111, 112-4, 216
    marital status and 116-7, 121, 123
    menopausal status and 44-66
    menstrual coping and 123
    oestrogen deficiency and 4-6, 13-5
    oestrogen replacement and 18-31
    psychosocial change and 102-15
    rating of 172
    role and status and 150-2, 212-4
    social class and 116, 118-9, 124-31, 212-4
    social deprivation and 157-60
    social network and 106
    social support and 205-6
    surveys of 44-71
    vulnerability and 199-208, 210-9

Cultural stability 153-7

Cultural variation in
    attitude to menopause 147-50, 153, 157
    behaviour at menopause 146-7
    child bearing role 149-52
    effects of employment 154-5
    role and status 150-7, 212-4
    social deprivation 157-60
    sociocultural stability 153-7
    symptoms 151-7

Definitions
   conceptual 8-10
   operational 167-9

Departure of children 103-15

Depression 92-7

Domino effect 33

Educational level 116-7, 121-3

Employment 116, 120-1, 127-31, 154-5, 214, 216

Empty nest 109-10

Exit stress 194-9

Factor analyses of
   attitudes 137
   symptoms 174-82

Hormones 2-3

International Health Foundation

   attitude survey 141-2
   symptom surveys 57-60, 75-9, 105-6, 123-9

Involutional melancholia 92-5

Life events during climacteric
   bereavement 199, 203-4
   a causal model of 206-8
   climacteric symptoms and 190-9
   cultural sensitivity to 203
   exit stress 194-9
   measurement of 187-90
   miscellaneous stress 194-9
   provoking agents 201-3, 207
   psychological symptoms and 192-4, 200
   social support and 205-6
   somatic symptoms and 192-4, 200, 204-6
   symptom formation factors 201
   types of life events 194-9
   types of symptoms and 197-9
   vulnerability factors 201-2, 207, 212

Marital relations 108, 111-4, 216

Marital status 116-7, 121, 123

Menopause
   age of 3-4
   conceptual definition 8-10
   hormones and 2-3
   operational definition of 50, 167-8
   ovarian failure and 2
   symptoms at 44-71

Menstrual coping 123

Mental tonic effect 33

Miscellaneous stress 194-9

Oestrogen deficiency
   atrophic vaginitis and 5
   ovarian failure and 2-3
   symptoms and 4-6, 13-5, 210
   vasomotor symptoms and 5-6

Oestrogen replacement
    atrophic vaginitis and 22, 25-8, 210
    controlled trials of 18-31
    domino effect 33
    early reports 15-7
    mental tonic effect 33
    personality and 34-5
    placebo effect of 31-2
    psychological symptoms and 32-3, 210
    psychological tests and 33-4
    psychotropic effects of 31-7, 210
    sexual functioning and 88-91
    vasomotor symptoms and 18-31, 210

Ovarian failure 2

Placebo effect 31-2

Provoking agents 201-3

Psychiatric disorders
    case definition of 97
    depression 92-7
    factor analyses of 94
    involutional melancholia 92-5
    risk at menopause 96
    surveys of 96-7

Psychosexual factors 83-7, 143-6

Psychosocial change
    empty nest 109-10
    loss of reproductive role 111, 144, 152, 212
    marriage of children 107-8
    maternal role 105-6, 111
    stages of child rearing 110, 112-4
    studies of 102-15
    theories of 101-2

Research methods
    assessment procedures 166
    conceptual definitions 8-11
    factor analyses 174-82
    operational definitions 167-9
    sample bias 165
    sample size 166
    symptom measurement 170-4, 183-5
    variation in 165

Role 150-7, 212-4

Self-esteem 216

Sexual functioning
    age and 80-5
    general population studies of 80-5
    hysterectomy and 86-8
    oestrogen replacement and 88-91
    oophorectomy and 86-8
    social factors and 83-5

Social class 116-9, 124-31, 213-4

Social deprivation 157-60

Social network 106

Social support 205-6

Status 150-7

Stereotype of menopause 141

Sociodemographic factors
    educational level and symptoms 116-7, 121-3
    employment and symptoms 116, 120-1, 127-31, 214
    income and symptoms 117, 123
    social class and symptoms 116-9, 124-31, 213-4

Symptom formation factors 201,

Symptoms (see climacteric symptoms)

Vasomotor instability 5-6

Vulnerability
    causal model of 206-8, 217-9
    climacteric 202, 210-1
    cultural factors and 203-4, 214-5
    factors determining 211-2
    life events and 199-208
    self-esteem and 216
    social role and 212-3
    social support and 205-6
    socioeconomic status and 213-4